Epidemiology Matters

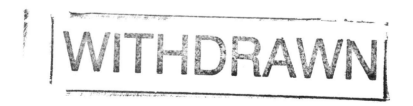

Epidemiology Matters

A New Introduction to
Methodological Foundations

KATHERINE M. KEYES

Department of Epidemiology, Columbia University

SANDRO GALEA

Department of Epidemiology, Columbia University

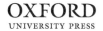

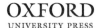

OXFORD
UNIVERSITY PRESS

Oxford University Press is a department of the University of
Oxford. It furthers the University's objective of excellence in research,
scholarship, and education by publishing worldwide.

Oxford   New York
Auckland   Cape Town   Dar es Salaam   Hong Kong   Karachi
Kuala Lumpur   Madrid   Melbourne   Mexico City   Nairobi
New Delhi   Shanghai   Taipei   Toronto

With offices in
Argentina   Austria   Brazil   Chile   Czech Republic   France   Greece
Guatemala   Hungary   Italy   Japan   Poland   Portugal   Singapore
South Korea   Switzerland   Thailand   Turkey   Ukraine   Vietnam

Oxford is a registered trademark of Oxford University Press
in the UK and certain other countries.

Published in the United States of America by
Oxford University Press
198 Madison Avenue, New York, NY 10016

Library of Congress Cataloging-in-Publication Data
Keyes, Katherine M., author.
Epidemiology matters : a new introduction to methodological foundations / Katherine M. Keyes, Sandro Galea.
   p. ; cm.
Includes bibliographical references.
ISBN 978-0-19-933124-6 (alk. paper)
I. Galea, Sandro, author.   II. Title.
[DNLM: 1. Epidemiologic Methods.   2. Epidemiologic Research Design.   3. Epidemiology. WA 950]
RA652.2.C55
614.4—dc23   2014001646

9 8 7 6 5 4 3
Printed in the United States of America
on acid-free paper

We dedicate this book to our families, who make our work worthwhile.

Contents

About the Authors

Katherine M. Keyes, PhD, is Assistant Professor of Epidemiology at Columbia University. Her research focuses on life course epidemiology with particular attention to psychiatric disorders, including cross-generational cohort effects on substance use, mental health, and chronic disease. She has particular expertise in the development and application of novel epidemiological methods and in the development of epidemiological theory to measure and elucidate the drivers of population health.

Sandro Galea, MD, DrPH, is Chair of the Department of Epidemiology at Columbia University. His work focuses on the social production of health of urban populations, innovative cells-to-society approaches to population health, and advancing a consequentialist approach to epidemiology in the service of population health. He is a past president of the Society for Epidemiologic Research and an elected member of the Institute of Medicine of the National Academies of Science.

Acknowledgments

THIS BOOK COULD not have been completed without the invaluable assistance of numerous students and colleagues. This book stands on the shoulders of many epidemiology and population health texts that we consulted throughout the writing of *Epidemiology Matters*. In particular, the writing of Raj Bhopal, Leon Gordis, Sander Greenland, Anwer Khurshid, Ollie Miettenen, Kenneth Rothman, Hardeo Sahai, Rodolfo Saracci, and Sharon Schwartz have not only been instructive but have provided invaluable guidance on how to present and formalize epidemiologic methods. In particular, discussions of epidemiologic methods with Sharon Schwartz have informed the structure and content of this text. Angelina Caruso was the architect of our hypothetical population of Farrlandians and provided editorial assistance on all aspects of the book. Sabrina Hermosilla provided valuable feedback on all of the text and figures and assisted with numerical examples. Linda Kahn assisted with exercises and problem sets for each of the chapters and provided keen editorial insight on the text. Adam Ciarleglio provided biostatistical expertise and editing throughout. All errors and omissions in this book are ours alone. Many of these chapters were piloted in two introductory epidemiology classes: Principles of Epidemiology at Columbia University, and the Epidemiology Core class at the *École des hautes études en santé publique* in Paris, France. We would like to thank Silvia Martins and Moise Desvarieux for allowing us to use the draft chapters in their courses and for their feedback on the chapters throughout the semester. We would also like to thank the students in these courses for valuable feedback. This book was primarily written during evenings, weekends, and even during vacations. We would like to thank our families for patiently allowing us the time and space to complete this text and for their encouragement and support along the way. Specifically, KMK would like to thank Jeff and Aidan Wild, and SG would like to thank Margaret Kruk, Oliver Luke Galea, and Isabel Tess Galea.

Prefatory Note

THIS BOOK SHOULD be read and used in conjunction with material available through our digital space: www.epidemiologymatters.org.

"Epidemiology Matters," the digital space, is intended to engage readers and learners on a continuum of instruction of ever-advancing epidemiologic methods. Here students and instructors will find material, topics, and examples that expand on the text in each of the chapters and material that complements text in the book. We also provide exercises and practice sets for each of the chapters and slide sets that can be used by lecturers. Answer keys for all exercises are available to instructors by emailing Katherine M. Keyes (kmk2104@columbia.edu) or Sandro Galea (sg22@columbia.edu). Further, we will regularly update the digital space with additional topics that were not covered in this text. Epidemiologymatters.org also provides additional instructional material on a wide variety of epidemiology and population health topics as a resource for researchers and lay professionals interested in developing skills in quantitative population health science.

Epidemiology Matters

1

An Introduction

EPIDEMIOLOGY IS THE science of understanding the causes and distribution of population health so that we may intervene to prevent disease and promote health. The definition of epidemiology has not substantially changed since the formal origins of the field more than 150 years ago (*Transactions of the Epidemiological Society of London*, 1876). Centrally there are, and have always been, two core functions for the field: (a) identifying causes of population health (b) so that we may intervene (Galea, 2013). These two core functions posit a pragmatic vision for the discipline: Epidemiology is the science of population health, aiming to understand the key causes of health and disease and doing so in a way that it may inform intervention so we may act.

The combination of scientific inquiry and call to action makes epidemiology a unique science. Identifying the causes of population health requires an understanding of the nature of populations; the conditions that shape them over time and place; and the policies, politics, and practices that create these conditions. With an eye toward the second part of the disciplinary definition, epidemiology focuses on asking questions that matter for the health of populations. As epidemiologists, we should be finding the answers that lead to conditions that shape healthy populations; we should be interested in an epidemiology of consequence (Galea, 2013). This, in our assessment, is a discipline worth getting excited about.

This is a dynamic time for epidemiology. In a time of dramatic population change, digital technology is rapidly making the world smaller and travel has become commonplace; ensuing changes in patterns of population interaction and behavior influence disease transmission. We are, for the first time, living in a predominantly urbanized world, with urban conditions influencing the water we drink, air we breathe, and how we think, feel, and behave; and the need for epidemiology has never been greater. The pressing health challenges of our time make the need for well-trained epidemiologists and public health professionals exigent. In this book, we aim to guide the reader toward an intuitive understanding of how the science of epidemiology can help us meet our mission: to understand the distributions and causes of disease that set the stage for us to act.

The Evolution of Epidemiology as a Discipline

The concept of epidemiology as a discipline of science is relatively recent, although the practice of conducting epidemiologic studies has had a much longer history. The methods by which we practice epidemiology have expanded with the development of the discipline itself. Many of the design and analytic techniques aimed at isolating and explaining the causes of disease arose in direct response to health concerns that arose during the 19th and 20th centuries. We refer readers to other works that much more fully summarize the history of epidemiology and emerging concepts in the field (e.g., Morabia, 2004).

By way of brief summary, the roots of epidemiology as a population health science can be traced to the 17th century, as John Graunt pioneered approaches to tabulating population health and mortality by presenting rates, ratios, and proportions of various causes of mortality. Epidemiologic science developed further in the 18th and 19th centuries as public health scientists such as William Farr developed more sophisticated life table approaches to understanding the force and burden of mortality, formally separated risks and rates, and luminaries such as John Snow used epidemiologic approaches to understand the London cholera epidemic. The basic measures of disease frequency and occurrence were all developed and applied to the prevailing public health problems of the time.

At the end of the 19th century much of the focus of public health and epidemiology was on infectious disease. This changed in the 20th century as antibiotics and broad adoption of hygiene and infection control contributed to a dramatic decrease in the burden of infectious diseases. Public health attention in high-income countries then shifted toward noncommunicable diseases and efforts to understand the causes of these diseases. With the advent and development of large-scale prospective studies in the mid-20th century, methods were needed to account for differential follow-up periods, exposure time, time-varying exposures, and competing risks. Concepts such as person time and differential loss to follow-up started receiving substantial attention in the literature, and methods became more formalized for the field in the 1970s (Steven & Laudan, 2013). In the 1980s, the advent of modern epidemiology, emerging through methodological work prominently including but not limited to Miettinen, Rothman,

Greenland, and others (Miettinen, 1985; Rothman & Greenland, 1998), helped formalize many of our central principles, providing insights such as the now commonplace understanding of case-control studies as sampling controls from the same source population as cases.

At the turn of the 21st century, two movements further broaden our conceptual lens. First, a set of theories articulated an ecosocial perspective on population health, which suggested that policies, institutions, and characteristics of context all contribute to the shaping of health (Krieger, 1994, 2012). The ecosocial perspective, combined with a tremendous increase in our understanding of variation in human biology—including how the human genome and epigenetic changes influence health and disease—has further afforded us the capacity to incorporate factors across levels to understand the production of health and disease. Second, we began to understand that the determinants of good health are distributed across the life course (Kuh, Ben-Shlomo, Lynch, Hallqvist, & Power, 2003), and in some cases, even before conception (Li, Langholz, Salam, & Gilliland, 2005). This suggests that to identify the causes of health and disease with the greatest actual impact on the health of the public, it is incumbent on the epidemiologist to conceptualize health across levels, across systems, and across the life course.

Therefore, at this writing early in the 21st century, we have come as a field to understand the causes of population health across levels of influence—from cells to society—and across the life course. Our methods have evolved and continue to evolve. And yet, despite the growth in our understanding of causes of health both in the broader social and contextual environment and across the life course, the fundamental study design and analysis issues articulated by our predecessors and advanced by our contemporaries remain the bedrock of good epidemiologic practice. Without a solid foundation in the fundamentals of epidemiologic design and analysis, there will be little learned from data collected cross-nationally and across biological systems. In this book, we aim to provide the reader with that foundation, applicable as much today as we hope it will be in coming decades as unforeseen changes challenge the scope of the discipline.

Our Approach to Teaching Epidemiology

We focus this book on the foundations of epidemiologic study design and basic analysis, informed by both classical and modern methodology. Our approach is also informed broadly by disciplines of clinical medicine, social science, philosophy, and statistics. At its core, we focus on an epidemiology that is consequential for the improvement of human health through the identification of causes of disease, always keeping an eye toward prevention and intervention. We do not focus on labeling key epidemiologic concepts in a specific sequence in an attempt to explain them. Our experience is that typically students memorize the rules and labels to understand the appropriate ways to conduct a study and draw inference. In this book, we aim to do things a bit differently and rest on the premise that the foundational concepts in epidemiology should be taught in a way that begins with the problems that motivate certain concepts; follows through with the connections among various concepts; and in the end, labels the concept after students fully understand the theory and rationale behind the method or methods in question.

Seven Steps in Conducting an Epidemiologic Study of Consequence

We have articulated our approach to teaching the basics of epidemiology around seven steps (see Box 1.1), with our chapters building on each step. Broadly, these steps involve defining a population of interest; identifying and developing measures of key health indicators and their potential determinants; taking a sample; estimating measures of health indicator occurrence, frequency, and association; and rigorously assessing internal validity, interactions, and external validity of the observed associations. We could devote an

---

BOX 1.1

Seven Steps for an Epidemiology of Consequence

Step 1: Define the population of interest

Step 2: Conceptualize and create measures of exposures and health indicators

Step 3: Take a sample of the population

Step 4: Estimate measures of association between exposures and health indicators of interest

Step 5: Rigorously evaluate whether the association observed suggests a causal association

Step 6: Assess the evidence for causes working together

Step 7: Assess the extent to which the result matters—is externally valid—to other populations

entire textbook to each one of these steps—in fact, many excellent texts are available that provide much greater detail on each step than we cover in this overview introductory book. Our purpose in explicating these steps is to concretize the basics of conducting an epidemiologic study, providing introductory students with a broad framework to understand the basics of our science by focusing on foundational concepts.

We begin with a focus on descriptive epidemiology, proceeding with Steps 1 to 4 of our seven-step series. We first illustrate how to define a population of interest. Even in this first step, there is substantial debate in the epidemiologic methods literature about how to define a population of interest and what should be included in this definition. We approach defining a population of interest through precise eligibility criteria focused on time and place, characteristics of individuals, and promotion of successful study completion and follow-up. We then focus on conceptualizing and measuring exposure and health indicators within that population. Next, we guide students through taking a sample of that population. Because we focus on an epidemiology of consequence for population health, we guide students through both representative samples of populations as well as purposive samples that are not representative but are instead designed to answer specific causal questions. We introduce students to basic epidemiologic study designs, including sampling individuals without the health indicator of interest and following them forward in time; taking snapshots of the population at a single point in time and estimating the prevalence of health indicators as well as concurrent associations with key potential determinants of interest; as well as sampling individuals with and without the health indicator of interest to compare exposure profiles. We also provide an overview of basic measures of association that quantify the effects of exposures on health indictors such as disease and illness.

After fully articulating foundational concepts in descriptive epidemiology, we then devote three full chapters solely to Step 5. Here we move from estimating associations to rigorously assessing those associations for causal effects. We do so by first presenting a theoretical framework for understanding causal effects, which is rooted in the counterfactual framework and informed by sufficient-component cause theory and life course theory. Once students have a grounded theoretical understanding of a cause, we present three chapters that articulate how noncausal associations arise in our data and what we can do to control for the effects of noncausal factors in the estimation of exposure-health indicator relations. We concatenate all noncausal factors into one rubric of non-comparability: That is, noncausal associations arise when exposed and unexposed individuals are not comparable on factors that cause disease and illness, and thus we articulate an organizing framework for understanding this phenomenon. We then explain how these noncausal associations arise—either by random chance, through measurement error, through selection, or through the association of causes with each other in the population of interest. After explaining how non-comparability arises, we articulate three fundamental ways in which we solve problems of non-comparability—stratification, randomization, and matching. We refer to related terms such as confounding and bias, but use the terms sparingly, as the distinction between confounding and bias can be quite arbitrary and the end result is often non-comparability regardless of the term that one uses.

Finally, we explore Steps 6 and 7 in Chapters 11 and 12. We focus on how to conceptualize and test for interactions between the exposure of interest and other potential exposures. An epidemiology of consequence is typically not interested in assessing the causal effect of a single exposure alone; we acknowledge that exposures are embedded in complex networks of biological and social influences that together produce adverse health for populations. Thus, an introductory understanding of how to assess causes working together (Chapter 11) can prepare the novice epidemiology student for conducting epidemiologic studies that move beyond the contribution of single exposures. We then devote a chapter (Chapter 12) to understanding external validity—the populations, places, and time periods in which the effects observed in a particular epidemiologic study apply outside of the particular study population to which the results are inferred. Finally, we present basic concepts in screening (Chapter 13), which aim to enable the student to understand one way in which we move forward to intervene and prevent disease.

Some steps are more involved than others. For example, we devote one chapter to taking a sample (Chapter 4), but three chapters (Chapter 8–10) to rigorously assessing whether an association is causal. Each step, however, is necessary for conducting an epidemiology of consequence with the explicit goal of improving population health. We recognize that some aspects of this framework are atypical for epidemiology textbooks. For example, few epidemiology textbooks focus on external validity and measurement; these concepts are more commonly found in textbooks on social science research methods. However, we have come to think that this framework provides an immensely organizing architecture both for how we may think of study validity in epidemiology and enables us to think of measurement, internal validity, and external validity among other areas of scientific study as part of a suite of epidemiologic approaches that are essential to robust causal thinking.

The Hypothetical Geographic Area of Inquiry: Farrlandia

Many of the examples in this book are based on a hypothetical geographic area that we term Farrlandia—a nod to the great epidemiologist and statistician, William Farr. We do this for several reasons. Most fundamentally, we want students to focus on the concepts that we are articulating rather than the specifics of a particular study. Use of hypothetical examples allows us to control the information and generate measures and associations that illustrate our concepts clearly. We can create examples that illustrate one principle at a time, rather than having to deal with the myriad of issues that arise in actual epidemiologic studies that complicate interpretation. Thus, we invite students into our world of Farrlandia in which diseases occur at a frequency that may not generalize to real populations but rather allows for clear instruction and interpretation of our basic principles.

Summary

A systematic grounding in the theoretical underpinnings of epidemiology as well as awareness of practical considerations are essential for any public health professional undertaking an epidemiologic study. In this text we aim to establish such a foundation by building on the methodological innovation and teaching of the previous century to provide introductory students with a systematic overview of how to understand the distribution and determinants of health and disease in populations. We present this introduction in a logical sequence aimed at explaining the foundations of how health and disease arise in populations and how we measure and count cases. We believe this approach will lead the next generation of public health, medical, and other professionals to a better understanding of our field and a richer understanding of the study designs and concepts that guide us toward identification of causes and ultimately prevention of disease and illness.

References

Transactions of the Epidemiological Society of London: Sessions 1866 to 1876: Objects of the Epidemiological Society. (1876). London: Epidemiological Society of London for the Investigation of Epidemic Diseases.

Galea, S. (2013). An argument for a consequentialist epidemiology. *American Journal of Epidemiological Study, 178*, 1185–1191.

Krieger, N. (1994). Epidemiology and the web of causation: Has anyone seen the spider? *Social Science and Medicine, 39*, 7, 887–903.

Krieger, N. (2012). Methods for the scientific study of discrimination and health: An ecosocial approach. *American Journal of Public Health, 102*, 936–944.

Kuh, D., Ben-Shlomo, Y., Lynch, J., Hallqvist, J., & Power, C. (2003). Life course epidemiology. *Journal of Epidemiological Community Health, 57*, 778–783.

Li, Y. F., Langholz, B., Salam, M. T., & Gilliland, F. D. (2005). Maternal and grandmaternal smoking patterns are associated with early childhood asthma. *Chest, 127*, 1232–1241.

Miettinen, O. (1985). *Theoretical epidemiology.* Albany, NY: Delmar Publishers, Inc.

Morabia, A. (2004). *A history of epidemiologic methods and concepts.* Boston, MA: Birkhauser Verlag.

Rothman, K. J., & Greenland, S. (1998). *Modern epidemiology.* Philadelphia: Lippincott-Raven.

Steven, H. W., & Laudan, A. (2013). *U.S. health in international perspective: Shorter lives, poorer health.* Washington, DC: The National Academies Press.

2

What Is a Population and What Is Population Health?

AS DEFINED IN Chapter 1, epidemiology is the science of understanding the causes and distribution of population health so that we may intervene to prevent disease and promote health. To practice epidemiology, the first step is to conceptualize, define, and operationalize what we mean by populations and population health. To understand this, we begin simply. The health indicators that matter for public health ultimately occur in individuals. Individuals, not populations, become ill, and much of clinical medicine is concerned with understanding why individuals become ill and how to treat illnesses. As shown in Figure 2.1, we have two individuals in our fictional population of Farrlandia, one of whom has a disease of interest to us (Individual A), one of whom does not (Individual B). The X on Individual A's chest marks disease. We can certainly ask questions about why Individual A became diseased, whereas Individual B was spared. We can examine their clinical and personal histories for clues and attempt to use inductive reasoning to discern the reasons that Individual A became diseased.

If we take a step back from individual cases, we can also conceptualize groups of individuals, some of who are ill and some of who are not. In Figure 2.2, we show 100 individuals, 20 of whom have disease and 80 of whom do not. Now, a different set of questions opens up to us. First, we can ask whether this disease is common or rare, what proportion of individuals is affected, and whether this disease represents a threat to the health of the

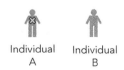

Individual
A

Individual
B

FIGURE 2.1 Two individuals, one diseased one not.

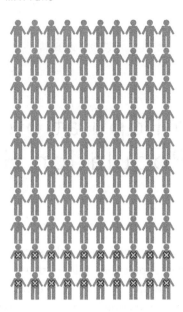

FIGURE 2.2 A set of 100 individuals, 20 of whom have disease.

population. Second, we can ask whether there are factors that are common among the 20 diseased compared with the 80 who are nondiseased, and if so, whether we can intervene on those factors to prevent future cases.

We take an even larger step back and compare three different sets of 100 people, as in Figure 2.3. On the left is the same set from Figure 2.2, with 20 diseased and 80 nondiseased people (we call them Set 1). In the center (Set 2) is a set with 5 diseased and 95 nondiseased people. On the right (Set 3) is a set with 60 diseased and 40 nondiseased people. This comparison now opens an even larger set of questions. Why is the disease relatively uncommon in Set 2, but very common in Set 3? What are the overarching factors that shape the distribution of the disease differently across these sets? Are the same factors more common among those with disease than those without in each of these sets?

The practice of epidemiology as a population health science asks these broader questions about the distribution of health and illness across sets of people—which we call *populations*. Populations can be defined in many ways that will be determined by the type of questions asked and the answers needed. Ultimately, we engage in this endeavor so that we can return to Figure 2.1 and understand why illness occurs in individuals. In Box 2.1 in the online material that accompanies Chapter 2, we provide additional insight into this issue by reviewing Geoffrey Rose's seminal paper on population health, "Sick Individuals and Sick Populations" (Rose, 1985).

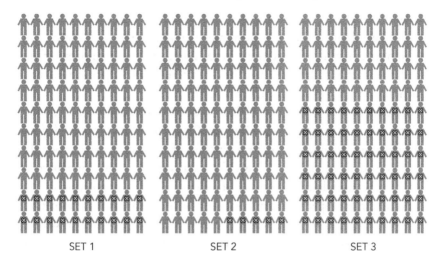

FIGURE 2.3 Three sets of 100 individuals.

Defining a Population of Interest

There are many ways in which a population of interest may be conceptualized and understood because there are many possible populations. In this section, we detail several dimensions through which we should conceptualize populations for the study of population health. Principally, populations are defined by eligibility criteria, that is, the characteristics of individuals in the population that make them of interest for epidemiological inquiry. Individuals may be eligible at one time and not eligible at another time. Populations that are defined in a way that individuals move in and out of eligibility are often termed dynamic populations; those in which individuals are either eligible or not, with no movement in and out, are termed stationary populations. These characteristics of the population of interest, including whether it is dynamic or stationary (see Box 2.2 of the online materials for Chapter 2), have implications for the analysis, interpretation, and generalizability of the results derived from studies of any particular population.

Setting Up Eligibility Criteria to Define the Population of Interest

Populations are collections of individuals within moments in time defined by at least one but potentially many organizing characteristics; these organizing characteristics form the eligibility criteria of the study. Eligibility criteria can be based on geographic area, time period, or characteristics of persons.

Depending on the research question of interest for which one initiates a study, the eligibility criteria may be minimal or quite extensive. Regardless of the number or nature of eligibility criteria, a fundamental component of any population health study is to define the characteristics of the population from which individuals will be drawn for the study.

There are three main categories that are commonly used to define the eligibility criteria of a population of interest. First, a population can be defined in terms of geographic area and time period of interest. Second, a population can be defined in terms of specific characteristics, events, or exposures for which health-related factors are of interest. Third, a population can be defined in terms of specific factors that promote successful study completion. It is worth noting that these eligibility categories are not mutually exclusive, and a single population may be defined using categories from all three criteria.

Types of Populations of Interest: Defined by Geographic Space and Time

Many public health questions require geographically defined populations. Local public health departments, for example, are charged with providing information on the distributions of specific health indicators in the catchment area of interest. We may be interested in estimating the burden of specific health indicators in a specific village, city, or country in a specific year or set of years. We also may be interested in the cases of a specific health indicator attributable to a certain exposure that is common in a particular geographic area.

Populations that are defined by time and place are often dynamic in nature. By dynamic, we mean that across time there are individuals entering and leaving the population, such that the actual composition of the population is changing. Consider the people in our fictional population of Farrlandia, shown in Figure 2.4.

In January of 2012, there are 100 individuals in our population. Over the course of 1 year, 28 individuals enter the population, through either birth or immigration from another geographic area. Over the same time period, 15 individuals leave the population, through either death or emigration out of the geographic area. Thus, in January 2013, there are 113 people in the population. Any population defined by eligibility criteria that allow movement in and out will have dynamic properties.

Understanding the characteristics across populations defined by geographic time and space is critical for many public health questions. This has

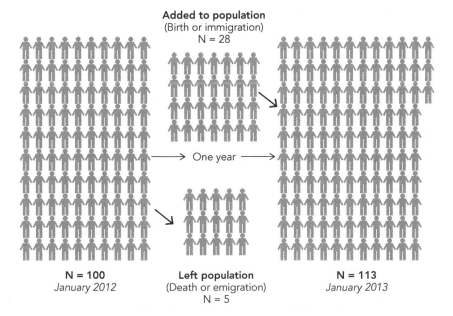

Added to population
(Birth or immigration)
N = 28

One year

Left population
(Death or emigration)
N = 5

N = 100
January 2012

N = 113
January 2013

FIGURE 2.4 Dynamic population of Farrlandia over 1 year.

perhaps been no more powerfully demonstrated than with studies showing that birth cohorts (groups of individuals defined by having been born in a certain year or set of years) often exhibit similarities in health across the span of their life courses and differences in health compared with individuals who are alive at the same time but have been born in different years (Finch & Crimmins, 2004; Kermack, McKendrick, & McKinlay, 2001).

Because populations defined by time and geographic space are often dynamic in nature, with individuals moving in and out of the population as defined by the particular eligibility criteria we are interested in, we can conceptualize these populations as being comprised not of people, but of lengths of eligible person time. We return to the concept of person time in Chapter 5, but we can intuitively understand the concept of person time by considering dynamic populations. Individuals only contribute information about the population during the time in which they are eligible. For example, suppose an individual moved to New York City from Toledo, lived in New York City for 2 years, and then moved to San Francisco. If we are interested in the health of New Yorkers, we can consider this individual has having contributed 2 years of his life (2 person years) to being eligible for understanding the health of New Yorkers. We can consider the individuals in the population as collections of eligible person time rather than collections of eligible people per se.

Types of Populations of Interest: Defined by a Characteristic, Event, or Exposure

Whereas many public health interests are defined by improving the health of individuals within a certain geographic area or certain time period, others may be defined by understanding the health of individuals possessing a certain characteristic or exposed to a certain event. For example, we may be interested in understanding the determinants of neonatal health, which would mean the population of interest would include newborn infants. The defining event for inclusion in the population of interest in this case is date of birth. Eligible individuals for our population may be those within a year of their birth. Other populations that may be of public health interest and defined by a specific event include pregnant women, individuals over the age of 65, individuals exposed to a natural or man-made disaster, individuals of certain races or ethnicities, individuals subject to particular laws, and many other potential characteristics.

Note that a geographic or temporal specifier need not define these populations for which eligibility is defined by particular characteristics. However, geographic or temporal specifiers may improve the clarity of the population definition. For example, if we are interested in health outcomes among pregnant women, we need to ask whether we are interested in all pregnant women or just pregnant women in a certain time period or geographic location. The research question largely dictates the population of interest. For example, if we are interested in how smoking during pregnancy affects neonatal health, we do not necessarily care where the pregnant women live or when they were pregnant. However, if we are interested in neonatal outcomes after the introduction of a program to enhance smoking cessation efforts among pregnant women in California, we would want to include a temporal and geographic specifier on the population of interest.

By way of illustration, a study conducted after the attack on the World Trade Center in 2001 examined neonatal outcomes among offspring of women in California who gave birth 6 months after the attack, compared with women who gave birth 6 months before the attack (Lauderdale, 2006). Offspring of Arab American women had lower birth weight 6 months after the attack than 6 months before the attack. This reduction in birth weight was not observed for other race or ethnicity groups. Thus, the population of interest for the study was defined by an event or exposure (pregnancy), a geographic location (California), and a time period (6 months before and after September 11, 2001).

Further, populations defined by a characteristic, event, or exposure can be dynamic as well. For example, if the population of interest is individuals aged 20–40 over the course of a several-year period of time, then the population will be dynamic because individuals will either become eligible when they turn 20 years old or no longer be eligible when they turn 41. Thus, even when the population is defined by events, characteristics, or exposures, we can still conceptualize the individuals who contribute to the population of interest as providing a collection of time during the period in which they meet eligibility criteria.

Types of Populations of Interest: Defined by Considerations of the Study

Finally, the population of interest may be a select group collected specifically to achieve a successful study. That is, we may define eligibility criteria such that we can be sure that the study participants will be good responders to our surveys or likely to continue to attend the health facility for follow-up visits. We may deem eligible individuals to be those who are relatively healthy so that they are unlikely to die during the course of the study from a health indicator that is outside the scope of our inquiry. Many clinical trials of new pharmaceutical medications, for example, include specific and numerous eligibility criteria to promote a successful study. Consider the Women's Health Initiative, a large study to assess the health benefits and risks of hormone replacement therapy after menopause (Writing Group for the Women's Health Initiative, 2002). Not only was eligibility limited to women who had undergone menopause, but researchers also excluded women with a history of certain medical conditions, women who were unlikely to be adherent to the study protocol, as well as women who failed to meet other criteria. Thus, the population of interest is a select subset of individuals defined not only by certain characteristics such as sex and menopausal status but also by other eligibility criteria that were introduced to achieve a more successful study to answer an etiological question.

We contrast the typical eligibility criteria defined to promote a successful study with those that are defined by geographic area and time. For example, when we ask questions about whether a certain drug works to prevent or delay a specific disease or other health indicator, we are not concerned with whether the new drug works among New Yorkers, or Californians, or during a specific time period. Rather, we are interested in forming a population base that is defined by specific and stringent eligibility criteria that allow for a precise answer to a specific etiological question about the efficacy of a new drug. The natural question that arises in that circumstance is the extent to which the findings from a study in which the eligibility criteria are defined to ensure a successful study will apply in other populations that are defined by other eligibility criteria that involve time and place. This process is termed the external validity of the study, and we cover this in Chapter 12.

Dynamic Versus Stationary Populations

Populations are inherently dynamic in nature. When we abstract a population for study, that population may remain dynamic or may become stationary due to the eligibility criteria that we set. Thus, we do not have a collection of individuals but rather a collection of eligible time contributed by each member of the population who meets the eligibility criteria for at least some period of time. Within the context of the particular study, the eligibility criteria can be defined such that the population is either dynamic or stationary. That is, studies with dynamic eligibility criteria for the population of interest include those that allow movement in and out. Populations with dynamic entry and exit are commonly those in which eligibility is defined by a time period and a geographic location. Stationary populations do not allow movement in and/or out. For example, if the population of interest is those who attended a church picnic, the population is stationary because eligibility criteria do not change over time; those who attended the church picnic are eligible for the study. Box 2.2 of the online materials that accompany this chapter summarizes dynamic versus stationary populations.

Summary

In epidemiology we are concerned with understanding the health of populations. Although illness ultimately occurs within individuals, epidemiologists ask questions about the health of groups, such as whether the illness is common or rare, why illness is more common in one group compared with another, and what the common causes of illness within a population of interest are. Defining a population of interest requires understanding several different dimensions, which we delineate by carefully considering eligibility criteria to set the frame of the population of interest. For example, we may be interested in the health of individuals who share a common geography, that is, who live in a certain area (village, city, country, etc.). We may also restrict the population to those who live in that area during a certain time period. Because populations dynamically flow in and out of populations, we can conceptualize the population of interest not as people per se but as the time that individuals contribute to the population of interest as eligible persons. Populations of interest can also be defined by certain characteristics such as being pregnant or newborn, within a certain age range, having a certain health condition, or having been exposed to a particular event of interest. Finally, we can also apply additional eligibility criteria to the population of interest to successfully achieve our research goals, such as ruling ineligible individuals with histories of certain health conditions or those who are unlikely to finish the study protocol. Regardless of the eligibility criteria that define the population of interest, the population may be dynamic or stationary, meaning that individuals recruited from the population base to the study may change over time depending on the eligibility criteria, and individuals may leave the population base as they die or no longer meet eligibility criteria. All of these factors together create a population base from which we can then conduct an epidemiologic study.

References

Finch, C. E., & Crimmins, E. M. (2004). Inflammatory exposure and historical changes in human life-spans. *Science, 305*(5691), 1736–1739.

Kermack, W. O., McKendrick, A. G., & McKinlay, P. L. (2001). Death-rates in Great Britain and Sweden: Some general regularities and their significance. *International Journal of Epidemiology, 30*, 678–683.

Lauderdale, D. S. (2006). Birth outcomes for Arabic-named women in California before and after September 11. *Demography, 43*, 185–201.

Rose, G. (1985). Sick individuals and sick populations. *International Journal of Epidemiology, 14*, 32–38.

Writing Group for the Women's Health Initiative. (2002). Risks and benefits of estrogen plus progestin in healthy postmenopausal women: Principal results from the Women's Health Initiative randomized controlled trial. *Journal of the American Medical Association, 288*, 321–333.

3

What Is an Exposure, What Is a Disease, and How Do We Measure Them?

EPIDEMIOLOGY AIMS TO document the health status of populations and to assess factors that cause poor health within and across populations so that we may intervene. In Chapter 2 we learned how to conceptualize populations and population health as emerging from the health status of individuals within the population and individuals contributing moments of eligible time to the particular population of interest for the study. In this chapter, we review how to conceptualize health status and common ways in which we measure the health status of populations; how to define exposures and other factors that may influence health; and several fundamental principles in the measurement of these factors.

What Is a Variable?

Throughout this book we discuss exposures, health indicators, and other health-related events, conditions, or states that differ across individuals in populations. We term all of the events, conditions, and states as variables. That is, a variable is any measured characteristic that differs across individuals. For example, age is a variable that we often use in epidemiology. Each individual in the population has an age, and not all individuals in the population have the same age. Sex, place of birth, occupation, cigarette smoking, diet, blood pressure, diabetes, pancreatic cancer, and any other measurable characteristic of individuals and their context are all potential variables that we may consider measuring in our epidemiologic studies.

What Are Health Indicators?

We are interested in the health of populations. Health can be conceptualized in many ways and is frequently defined, in epidemiology, by its absence. Therefore, we measure the presence of diseases in individuals, but we can also measure the occurrence of infections, syndromes, symptoms, and biological or subclinical markers associated with disease. We are interested in how these illnesses and symptoms affect individuals over the life course, with the disability that is associated with the presence of disease and the potential years of life lost due to the presence of illness. Conversely, we are also interested in health itself, measuring quality of life, wellness, and activity. In this book, we are broadly interested in health states and therefore we call the measures of health that are of interest to epidemiologists "health indicators." We do so to acknowledge that—as public health professionals—we are responsible for describing and understanding a vast array of potential illnesses and health states. As appropriate, we also at times refer to health states as outcomes, diseases, illnesses, and disease states.

To conduct epidemiologic studies, we need to measure health indicators as variables that are heterogeneous across individuals. There are several common ways in which health indicators are so measured. We review three common ways in which health indicator variables are measured: binary, ordinal, and continuous.

Binary Health Indicators

Many health indicators are typically conceptualized as present or absent; we consider a variable that takes on two values (in our case, presence or absence of disease) to be in binary categories. An individual either has a diagnosis of diabetes, cancer, Alzheimer's disease, or HIV or does not. We term health indicators that are measured as present or absent as binary variables. For pedagogical purposes, most of the examples that we use throughout this text will focus on binary indicators of the presence or absence of a health indicator.

Ordinal Health Indicators

Moving beyond the basic presence or absence of a particular disease or syndrome, ordinal health indicators can take on several graded values. These graded values are still categories; the difference between ordinal and binary indicators is that rather than two categories, there are more than two, and the ordering of the categories is meaningful. For example, a common if rudimentary way to estimate health in populations is to ask survey participants, "How would you rate your health?" Response options typically include excellent, good, fair, and poor. These response options are ordinal, or graded, because excellent health is better health than good and good is better health than fair, and so forth. However, importantly, although ordinal indicators imply a sequencing, they do not imply a consistent measurement of distance between response options. That is, we do not assume that "excellent" is exactly the same amount better than "good" as "fair" is better than "poor." This limits somewhat the utility of ordinal health indicators. Other types of ordinal health indicators include asking respondents how often they experience certain symptoms or states associated with adverse health. For example, we might be interested in how difficult it is for an individual to climb a flight of stairs, with response options including "Very difficult," "Somewhat difficult," and "Not difficult." Again, these options are graded because finding stair climbing very difficult indicates worse health than finding stair climbing somewhat difficult.

Continuous Health Indicators

Many indicators of health reflect a much wider range of variation than presence or absence or ordinal sequences. Diastolic and systolic blood pressure, cholesterol, viral load, cancer stage, and weeks of pregnancy are all measures of health that are represented continuously in the population with a wide range of values across individuals. Capturing and describing the health of populations requires assessment of this underlying continuous variation as well as the binary presence or absence of different health conditions. Continuous health indicators also include important concepts such as disability. Disability is typically conceptualized in a health context as a broad term encompassing any type of impairment or reduced functioning in daily life and may be due to symptoms or diseases. Disabilities are context dependent, as the reduction in functioning depends on environmental conditions and barriers.

What Is an Exposure?

In this book, we use an imperfect but practical term "exposure" to denote a wide range of variables that may cause health indicators or may be associated with variables that cause health indicators. The term exposure is used widely in epidemiology for this purpose. Exposure typically denotes contact with something that may be harmful. However, we use the term more broadly to denote any variable that may affect health or may be associated with health, either in a positive or a negative way. Exposures can range from the very macro social environment to the molecular level. For example, individuals are exposed to policies and laws within the society in which they live. These policies and laws may affect health in certain ways and as epidemiologists, it is our charge to study the ways in which these policies and laws impact health.

We do not necessarily imply a causal relation with health when we term a variable an exposure. Exposures are variables that we wish to evaluate for their potential relation with adverse health outcomes or variables that denote groups at particularly higher risk for adverse health. For example, we consider biological sex an exposure that may be associated with adverse health outcomes. Men on average die earlier than women and are more likely than women to die of cardiovascular disease. Women, on the other hand, are more likely than men to evince health indicators such as major depression and anxiety. We consider biological sex an exposure variable in the sense that it is a measureable characteristic of people that varies within a population and may be a useful descriptor of health states.

Exposures can also be described at the molecular level, such as particular genes, genetic variants, or genetic sequences that denote individuals who may have a predisposition for an adverse health outcome. The emerging field of epigenetics has also sparked interest in describing how social circumstances or other exposures can impact the way in which genetic sequences are expressed (Petronis, 2010). Neurological signals such as the activation of particular brain regions is another a source of variation that we can exploit for understanding the distribution and cause of health outcomes (Falk et al., 2013). All of these factors fall under the rubric of what we term exposures.

Our charge as epidemiologists is to accurately capture exposure over time. This is easier said than done. We must also contend with measurement issues and the analytic challenges that come with such exposure variability. We cover some of this in later chapters, but first here we discuss types of exposures and duration of exposures—two concepts that are central to our understanding of epidemiologic measurement.

Types of Exposures

Under the broad umbrella of exposures, there are many different ways in which exposures can be distributed both within an individual and across a population. In the following, we describe four important potential types of exposures that may be necessary for understanding health: (1) innate, (2) acute, (3) chronic or stable exposures, and (4) time-varying exposures.

Innate Exposures

Individuals are born exposed to certain factors such as their biological sex, race and ethnicity, and DNA sequence. They are present at birth and most often carried with individuals throughout the span of life. We also note that although we are born with characteristics such as biological sex and race, the relations between these exposures and health are often attributable to social factors—for example, discrimination, social position, and marginalization (Krieger, 2012). Thus, whereas biological sex and race are innate, there is not necessarily anything biologically programmed about the effects of these variables on health.

Acute Exposures

Acute exposures are exposures that occur for a relatively short duration and do not recur. Acute exposures may include such factors as the threat to physical integrity from natural or human-made disasters, exposures endured during the period of gestation, and sudden stressful situations or events that resolve quickly.

Chronic Exposures

Chronic exposures are those that do not change over time and may include factors such as pollution, poverty, neighborhood instability, and policies and laws. We differentiate between chronic exposures that are imposed from the environment in which one lives, such as pollution and poverty, from innate exposures such as biological sex and DNA. Although biological sex and DNA can be considered chronic exposures, they may be meaningfully different in terms of their relation with health from chronic exposures that occur outside of the set of factors that an individual is born with. Further, chronic exposures need not by definition be chronic; the majority of families who spend some time living in poverty, for example, will not spend their whole lives in poverty. Thus, a final category is necessary to describe the main ways in which exposures can be conceptualized: time-varying or dynamic exposures.

Time-Varying or Dynamic Exposures

Finally, many exposures are neither acute nor chronic, but vary across the life course of an individual. Diet, exercise, smoking, and alcohol consumption, for example, are well known to affect health, and often change within a person and across time.

For example, describing a woman as a smoker without qualification ignores the degree and intensity with which her smoking habits have potentially changed during her life. This individual may have started using cigarettes occasionally, begun using daily some time after, and stopped and started multiple times throughout her life. Although there are certainly individuals who, for example, smoke cigarettes consistently and heavily for many years (thus they would be chronically exposed), it is more common for individuals to change their cigarette consumption pattern over time with periods of abstinence, light use, and heavy use.

We also need to capture multiple dynamic exposures as they unfold. Consider the complexity in measuring two exposures—smoking and exercise—for four individuals in Farrlandia studied over 7 years, shown in Figure 3.1. Black denotes a time period in which an individual regularly smoked cigarettes and dots denote a time period in which an individual regularly exercised. Angelina smokes for the first 2 months of the study and then quits smoking and starts exercising through the remainder of the study. Todd was a nonsmoking regular exerciser throughout the entire 7 years of the study. Jose did not exercise at all and smoked regularly from Month 2 to Month 6. Ananda started the study as a nonsmoker, started smoking after 2 months, and remained a smoker for the rest of the study. Todd and Ananda developed cardiovascular disease, each

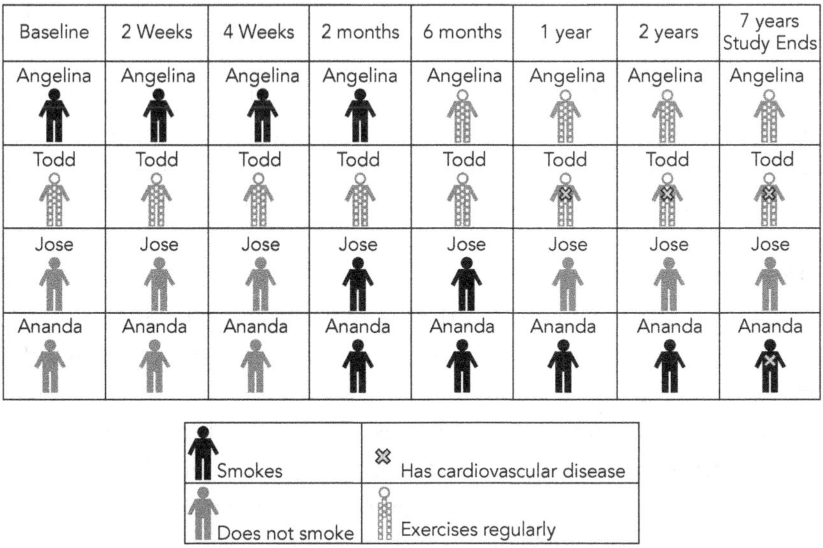

FIGURE 3.1 Smoking and exercise among five individuals in Farrlandia over time.

at a different time point. Our measurement of how exercise and smoking are associated with cardiovascular disease must take into account the time-varying nature of these exposures for some individuals in the study.

In summary, exposure is a term that is used to denote a wide range of potential variables that individuals in our population acquire. This may include variables that individuals are born with, such as genetic sequence and biological sex; social circumstances that may or may not change over the life course; acute exposures such as stressful events; and time-varying exposures such as diet and substance use.

Duration of Exposure, Latency, and Critical Windows

In addition to exposure to certain factors potentially varying across time, the effects of those exposures may also vary depending on the duration of exposure and on the period in the life course when one is exposed.

Duration of Exposure

For certain exposures, the duration of the exposure matters for the production of adverse health. Smoking a single cigarette is unlikely to have long-term health consequences, but smoking more than a pack of cigarettes per day for 40 years could result in some adverse health consequences. Similarly, one meal laden with trans-fat and calories is unlikely to cause heart disease, whereas the effects of years of unhealthy eating may accumulate to adversely impact health. Whether duration matters or not may depend on the health indicator of interest. For example, a single episode of extreme binge drinking (defined as 10 or more drinks in a single drinking episode; Patrick et al., 2013) may influence injury (e.g., alcohol poisoning, falls, motor vehicle crashes) but may not contribute to the development of cirrhosis. However, a long-term pattern of regular heavy and extreme alcohol consumption may influence the development of cirrhosis.

Latency and Critical Windows

The timing of the exposure across the life course may also be important for developing an accurate assessment of the impact of an exposure on health. One example of this is fetal exposures and later offspring health (Ben-Shlomo & Kuh, 2002). The period of gestation is a critical developmental window in which development of organs and neurological function is happening at a rapid and often exponential pace. Exposures that occur during gestational development can have immediate effects (e.g., heavy alcohol consumption in pregnancy is known to cause, in some circumstances, a syndrome at birth termed Fetal Alcohol Syndrome in offspring), but may also not manifest their effects for years or even decades. For example, extreme caloric restriction during the first trimester of fetal development is associated with the development of schizophrenia and related neurodevelopmental outcomes during adulthood (Susser & Lin, 1992). Beyond the neonatal period, child exposures such as maltreatment may affect health throughout the life course and may not manifest until adulthood (Heim & Nemeroff, 2001). Thus, there may be critical windows of development in which exposures have an effect on health indicators. Furthermore, these effects may not manifest for years or even decades after the exposure occurs, which is considered the latency period. In Box 3.1 of the online material that accompanies Chapter 3, we provide some additional empirical examples of how duration, latency, and critical windows vary across the life course in ways that may impact health indicators of interest. Careful conceptualization and measurement of the proper point in human development for which the exposures of interest may influence health indicators is critical if the effects of those exposures are to be observable.

An Introduction to Measurement of Exposure and Health Indicators

Once we have conceptualized the exposure(s) and health indicator(s) of interest for study, and the proper developmental window to assess exposures and latency period after which to capture the effects of the exposures, the next step is to decide how to measure these factors. Measurement is a rich and vibrant area of epidemiology, and good measurement of our variables of interest is critical if we want to draw any conclusions from an epidemiologic study. But what is good measurement? We discuss two fundamental ways in which we evaluate how good our measures are—the reliability of the measure and the validity of the measure.

We introduce these concepts through an example. Suppose that we would like to study whether individuals who have depression are more likely to develop overweight than individuals without depression. Depression is a condition characterized by disabling feelings of hopelessness, sadness, and loss of interest in activities. How should we measure this constellation of symptoms? We could simply ask people, "Are you depressed?" This is problematic for a number of reasons. Will those we ask know what we mean by "depressed"? Will individuals in the study understand the question and all interpret the question in the same way? What time frame are we interested in? Someone may feel sad today because they received bad news, but would not feel sad next week if asked the same question. Others may interpret the question more generally and tell us if they have been feeling depressed over the past month. Therefore, to avoid this confusion, we may want to ask respondents a series of questions that would measure several symptoms that could suggest depression and would be precise about the time frame of interest (e.g., "have you felt sad most of the day nearly every day over the past 2 weeks?"). Turning to obesity, what do we mean by obesity? Excess body weight for size? How should it be measured? Should we use the World Health Organization standard of a body mass index (BMI) of 30 or greater based on height and weight? High performance athletes often have high BMI without excess body weight for size, thus we may want to consider wait circumference, fat calipers, or bioelectrical impedance as our measure of obesity. If we use BMI, should we ask people their height and weight or use a ruler and a scale? What are the pros and cons of each approach? Figure 3.2 displays a list of questions that we should ask ourselves about our measures, corresponding to the sections following.

Be Clear About What Is Being Measured

A construct is an idea or theory of what we are interested in measuring, such as depression, obesity, or any other health indicator or exposure. The construct

What is the construct we wish to measure? Is it clear and specific?	Construct to be measured	
Propose item(s) that capture the construct. Are the measures easily interpretable, short, and clear?	Items attempting to measure the construct Item 1 Item 2 Item 3 Item 4	
Are the measures reliable? • Would the same person answer similarly when asked on two occasions? • Would two different raters judge the item the same way? • Are the items clustered together in terms of response?	Reliable Tightly clustered	Not reliable Loosely clustered
If measures are reliable, are they valid? • High sensitivity and specificity • Related to other measures that they should be related to • Unrelated to other measures that they should not be related to	Valid Hits the target	Not Valid Misses the target

FIGURE 3.2 Developing measures for epidemiologic investigation: Steps toward reliability and validity.

itself is distinct from the measurement of the construct. Our goal in measurement is to create tools that allow us to capture the underlying constructs that we wish to study as well as possible.

If Measurements Include Questions That Will Be Answered by Respondents, Make Sure Questions Are Easily Interpretable, Short, and Clear

Questions should be easily interpretable and clear for quality measurement. For example, when assessing depression, "In the past week, how often have you felt hopeless about the future?" would be a clearer question than, "In the past week, how often have you felt sad or hopeless?" The latter question combines two different symptoms: sadness, and hopelessness. Time frames should be carefully considered. Our example used "In the past week . . .", but we could assess symptoms of depression in the past month, year, or in the respondent's lifetime, among many other potential time frames.

The Measures Used Should Be Reliable

Reliability of a measure is the extent to which it is a consistent indicator of the construct of interest. In the following, we review three questions that address whether a measure is reliable.

Would the Respondent Answer the Question Similarly If Asked at Two Different Time Points?

One way we can estimate the reliability of a measure is to have a respondent answer the question or questions at two different time points. Assuming the underlying construct is invariant over time (i.e., there is no true change in the underlying construct), the respondent should answer the same way across time for the measure to demonstrate reliability. For example, suppose our construct of interest is literacy. We have respondents take a reading test, and then 1 week later we have them take the same test. To the extent that they score similarly on the reading test at the two time points, we would consider the reading test to be a reliable indicator of literacy. However, if the individual took reading classes over the week between tests, or remembered the test questions and then answered differently the second time, this would violate our measure of the reliability of the reading test, as there was true change between testing sessions. This is often termed test–retest reliability.

Would Two or More Judges Give the Respondent the Same Value?

When a rater judges the construct of interest, we can assess the reliability of the rater by having multiple, independent raters judge the same construct. For example, suppose we are conducting a study of cervical cancer. A pathologist will assess a cervical biopsy for the presence of cancerous cells. We can assess the reliability of having a single pathologist judge the biopsy by first conducting a study in which multiple pathologists rate the biopsy. For example, if we asked three pathologists to review the same cervical biopsy, would they all come to the same conclusion about the presence or absence of cervical cancer? If they agree, then using a single pathologist to diagnose cervical cancer based on a biopsy has good reliability; if not, then reliability is poor and another measure of cancer is needed. The process of having multiple raters judge the measure of the construct of interest is often termed inter-rater reliability.

If Multiple Items Are Generated, Do They Cluster Together?

Using multiple questions to measure the same underlying construct is an important way to achieve reliability of measurement. The process of creating and assessing the reliability of multiple measures of the same underlying construct is termed scale development (Brown, 2006; DeVellis, 2003; Shadish, Cook, & Campbell, 2002). We present here a brief introductory overview.

As the number of questions that attempt to tap into the same underlying construct increases, the reliability of the measurement of that construct should increase, to the extent that we are using questions that actually measure the construct itself. We can measure how reliable the multiple-question scale is at assessing the same underlying construct by examining how often, for example, individuals who were sad in the past week were also hopeless and thought about death frequently (i.e., how often these items cluster together within individuals). As the association between feeling sad, feeling hopeless, and having thoughts of death increases, the reliability of the three measures increases, as capturing the same underlying construct also increases. As we add more items that capture depressed mood, the reliability of the scale will also increase. There are two important caveats to this. First, if we include items that are not indicative of the underlying construct of depressed mood, then the reliability of our scale will decrease. Second, if we include items that are redundant with each other, then we may increase reliability but at the expense of efficiency. This process of assessing how closely items within a scale are associated with one another is often termed the internal consistency reliability.

Assess the Validity of the Measures

Even if we have very reliable measures of the constructs of interest, it is also important to assess the validity of the measures. By validity, we mean whether the measures actually capture the underlying construct of interest that we are intending to capture.

A measure cannot be valid if it is not reliable, but a reliable measure can be invalid. That is, we can reliably measure the wrong construct. The validity of a measure of exposure or health indicator is of principal importance when embarking on an epidemiologic study. Are we actually capturing individuals with the health indicator of interest? Are those we designate as exposed actually exposed? For example, suppose we are interested in studying the construct of intelligence as a health indicator among young adults. By intelligence, we are broadly interested in the ability to abstractly reason and use logic for problem solving. To measure intelligence among young adults, we use scores on a standardized test used for entrance into secondary education. These measures are very reliable and have high internal consistency and test–retest association. However, they may not be valid indicators of intelligence, as scores on a standardized test for entrance into secondary education are influenced by social context, test-taking ability, and preparation time. Thus, we have a reliable measure that may be invalid in capturing the construct of interest.

One way to conceptualize the relation between reliability and validity, as shown in Figure 3.2, is to conceptualize the construct as a target, with the items that are actually measured being points that may or may not hit the target. Thus, we can have measures that are reliable in that multiple raters rate them the same way, individuals respond similarly on more than one occasion, and the items tend to cluster together within individuals, but that do not in fact capture the actual construct we want to measure. We would say in that case that the items miss the target—they are not valid.

There are many different ways to calibrate the validity of a particular epidemiologic measure. As an introduction, we will review a fundamental way to conceptualize validity, which is through the sensitivity and specificity of the measure compared with a gold standard.

What is a Gold Standard?

We refer to a gold standard as the most reliable and valid known measure of the construct of interest. A gold standard could be a biomarker for the exposure or health indicator; a diagnosis or assessment from a trained and expert clinician; or any other measure that is the best-known indicator of the presence, absence, or degree of the construct of interest.

Although of course it would always be preferable to use the gold standard as a measure in an epidemiologic study, there are many different logistical and practical reasons why we might choose to use an alternative measure. For example, biological specimens or clinical assessment may be difficult or impossible to obtain depending on the study design and may be cost prohibitive for the whole study sample. Further, if there are less costly methods to obtain necessary information from participants with a similar degree of validity as a gold standard, then it may be more efficient for the study as a whole to use a measure that is not the gold standard. When possible, however, a new measure that is being considered should first be compared with the gold standard as a preliminary step before it is included in a larger epidemiologic study.

Sensitivity and Specificity Using a Gold Standard Comparison

If we have a gold standard for comparison, we can determine the proportion of people who are actually exposed (or actually have the health indicator in question) and who are correctly categorized as exposed using our measure, as well as the proportion of people who are actually unexposed and who are correctly classified as unexposed using our measure.

As an example, suppose that we want to assess the prevalence of smoking a pack or more of cigarettes per day within a population. We could ask members of the population, "In the past 24 hours, how many cigarettes have you smoked?" However, some people in the population may lie (given the social stigma associated with smoking), some people may not understand the question, and some people may overestimate or underestimate the number of cigarettes smoked. In general, there will be error in estimating pack-a-day smoking. We could, in a subsample of participants, use a blood sample to assess the blood level of cotinine, a biomarker for tobacco smoke exposure. The level of cotinine in the blood increases with exposure to more cigarette smoke, as it is an alkaloid found in tobacco smoke and retained in the blood stream with a half-life of about 20 hours. Cotinine levels above 300 ng/mL are indicative of heavy smoking, at least approximately a pack per day (20 cigarettes in standard packs). We could then measure the sensitivity of the self-report of smoking (given that you smoke a pack or more per day, what is the probability that you report smoking a pack or more per day) and the specificity of the self-report of smoking (given that you do not smoke, what is the probability that you report not smoking). In Box 3.2 of the online material that accompanies this chapter, we detail a quantitative example of sensitivity and specificity for measure validity. We also delve into greater detail on sensitivity and specificity in Chapter 13.

What Do We Do When There Is No Gold Standard?

For many of the measures that we are interested in for characterizing population health, there are no gold standards. Even with biomarkers, many have validity problems of their own and are thus not gold standards. Further, clinician diagnoses are often not reliable from clinician to clinician (Aboraya, Rankin, France, El-Missiry, & John, 2006), limiting their utility as gold standards. When gold standards are not available, there are many other options for validity analyses. Concurrent/predictive validity is one common approach to assessing validity when there is no gold standard. For a measure to have concurrent or predictive validity, it should be associated with other exposures and health indicators that the underlying construct is known to be associated with. For example, if our construct of interest is high cholesterol, our measure of cholesterol should be higher as the body mass index of our sample increases, given the ample epidemiologic evidence that average cholesterol increases with body size. Another approach to validity when there is no gold standard is an assessment of divergent validity. For a measure to have divergent validity, it should not be associated with other exposures and health indicators that the underlying construct of interest is not associated with. For example, there is no evidence to indicate that cholesterol is associated with color preferences. If we can demonstrate that cholesterol is not associated with color preference, we are increasing our assurance of the validity of the measure. The key to validity analysis is that it should be systematic and comprehensive and should use multiple types of analyses to triangulate on the validity or invalidity of the particular measure.

Summary

Conceptualization and measurement of health in populations is critical to the success of improving population health. Health indicators span a host of health-related phenomena, including the presence of disease, symptoms, syndromes, and disability as well as wellness, quality of life, and other health-related states. Potential influences on these health-related states can broadly be considered exposures, which include acute and chronic influences, health behaviors, genetic markers, and any other factors that vary within individuals, across individuals, and/or across populations. Exposures can be long or short in duration and may have an impact only at a critical point in human development. Conceptualizing a framework for understanding how key potential exposures of interest may influence health indicators of interest is vital for designing and conducting an epidemiologic study. Once a framework has been articulated, measures of health indicators and exposures must be created, with careful assessments of reliability and validity.

References

Aboraya, A., Rankin, E., France, C., El-Missiry, A., & John, C. (2006). The reliability of psychiatric diagnosis revisited: The clinician's guide to improve the reliability of psychiatric diagnosis. *Psychiatry (Edgmont)*, *3*(1), 41–50.

Ben-Shlomo, Y., & Kuh, D. (2002). A life course approach to chronic disease epidemiology: Conceptual models, empirical challenges and interdisciplinary perspectives. *International Journal of Epidemiology*, *31*, 285–293.

Brown, T. A. (2006). *Confirmatory factor analysis for applied research*. New York: Guilford Press.

DeVellis, R. F. (2003). *Scale development: Theory and applications*. Thousand Oaks, CA: Sage Publications.

Falk, E. B., Hyde, L. W., Mitchell, C., Faul, J., Gonzalez, R., Heitzeg, M. M. . . . Schulenberg, J. (2013). What is a representative brain? Neuroscience meets population science. *Proceedings of the National Academy of Sciences of the United States of America*, *110*(44), 17615–17622.

Heim, C., & Nemeroff, C. B. (2001). The role of childhood trauma in the neurobiology of mood and anxiety disorders: Preclinical and clinical studies. *Biological Psychiatry*, *49*, 1023–1039.

Krieger, N. (2012). Methods for the scientific study of discrimination and health: An ecosocial approach. *American Journal of Public Health*, *102*, 936–944.

Patrick, M. E., Schulenberg, J. E., Martz, M. E., Maggs, J. L., O'Malley, P. M., & Johnston, L. D. (2013). Extreme binge drinking among 12th-grade students in the united states: Prevalence and predictors. *JAMA Pediatrics*, *167*, 1019–1025.

Petronis, A. (2010). Epigenetics as a unifying principle in the aetiology of complex traits and diseases. *Nature*, *465*(7299), 721–727.

Shadish, W. R., Cook, T. D., & Campbell, D. T. (2002). *Experimental and quasi-experimental designs for generalized causal inference*. Boston: Houghton Mifflin.

Susser, E. S., & Lin, S. P. (1992). Schizophrenia after prenatal exposure to the Dutch Hunger Winter of 1944-1945. *Archives of General Psychiatry*, *49*, 983–988.

4

What Is a Sample?

WE HAVE NOW covered the first two steps of our seven-step approach: defining a population of interest and conceptualizing and creating measures of exposures and health indicators. Once we have accomplished these elements, the next step is to take a sample of the population and decide how to study that sample (i.e., follow people forward in time, take a snapshot of the population at a particular time, or sample people based on whether they have the outcome or not).

Most populations of interest for health, as noted in Chapter 2, are dynamic, with people moving into and out of the population constantly. Within the context of a dynamic population in which people are entering and exiting across time, how do we examine the potential causes that underlie health outcomes?

Why Take a Sample, and What Kind of Sample Is Appropriate for the Research Question?

Why do we take samples? If we epidemiologists had our way, we would study everybody, all the time. That means we would have a complete census of people, observe what they are exposed to and what diseases they develop, and take consistent and careful measurements at regular intervals. However, this is not possible, principally for pragmatic reasons—we rarely have the time and money to collect health information on everyone in a population, and even if we did, it would likely be a waste of resources. By carefully and correctly taking a sample of the underlying population we can often arrive at the same answer to the health-related research question that we would have arrived at by interviewing the whole population. Thus, we take samples because it is more efficient in terms of time and resources than collecting data on an entire population.

There are two key questions to wrestle with before we take a sample. First, we need to specify the population of interest; second, we to need to specify the research question of interest. We discuss each in turn.

Specifying a Population of Interest

We have reviewed principles for selecting a population of interest in Chapter 2. Without specifying a population of interest, there is no way to determine whether the sample chosen is appropriate for answering the research question of interest. A general method for selecting such a population is to ask, what are the characteristics of the population in which we would like to understand health? Do we want to know what the prevalence of diabetes is within New York City?, New York State?, The United States? Do we want to know the causes of diabetes? Each has different implications for how we would select a sample for robust inference.

We also note that populations of interest may be broader than collections of individuals. We may be interested in differences across cities, countries, or any other unit of measurement. For example, we may be interested in whether countries with different dietary norms have different rates of a certain health indicator compared with other countries, or whether cities that fluoridate water have different rates of dental cavities compared with cities that do not fluoridate water. Studies that have groups (e.g., counties, countries) as their unit of analysis are typically called "ecologic studies." Importantly, however, the study design considerations remain the same regardless of the unit of analysis in which we are interested.

Specifying the Research Question of Interest

The research question of interest will clarify what the appropriate way to sample from the population of interest will be. Although there are many different types of research questions, two that have major implications for study design are whether we are interested in (a) estimating population parameters or (b) estimating causal effects of exposures on outcomes. We separate these two types of research questions deliberately because the samples needed to answer these two questions are different.

One of the most fundamental roles of epidemiology is to document population parameters. Questions concerned with population parameters include, for example, "What proportion of individuals in the population of interest has breast cancer?" "What is the mean blood pressure in the population?" "How many new cases of HIV are diagnosed in the population over 3 years?" Population parameters include estimates of proportions, means and standard deviations, and other indicators of the health status of populations. We detail the estimation of these measures in Chapter 5. Of central concern, to estimate the distribution and burden of health indicators in the population, we need a representative sample of that population. By a representative sample, we mean that the sample taken has characteristics that are similar to the overall population, such that the mean blood pressure in the sample is similar to the mean blood pressure in the overall population.

Although we are interested in documenting the burden of disease in populations, we are also interested in understanding what causes adverse health outcomes. We detail a theoretical framework for causal inference in Chapter 7; but there are central questions for which these measures are needed such as "Does exposure to pollution cause lung cancer?" "Does suffering maltreatment in childhood cause depression in adulthood?" "Does prenatal exposure to smoking cause cognitive deficits in childhood and adulthood?" "Does a specific genetic marker cause Alzheimer's disease?" Note that these types of questions differ from questions around population parameters; we no longer want to estimate the proportion of the population that has a particular health outcome. Rather, we want to know whether there is a causal effect of a certain exposure or exposures on a particular health outcome or health outcomes.

When our central interest is in estimating causal effects, the principal concern in terms of sampling is not representativeness. The principal concern is whether individuals exposed to the hypothesized cause of interest are comparable with individuals who are not exposed. Comparability is a core concept in epidemiology. To determine whether an exposure has a causal effect on a health indicator, we need exposed and unexposed groups that are similar on all factors associated with the health indicator except for the exposure. We discuss the issue of comparability more comprehensively in Chapters 8–10. For this chapter, it is an important fundamental to recognize that in many cases we do not take representative samples of the population for epidemiologic studies; instead we take purposive samples to achieve comparability between groups of exposed and unexposed persons so that we can identify causes.

Representative samples and purposive samples are not necessarily mutually exclusive. In many cases we take a representative sample so that we can estimate population parameters and additionally design the study so that we can achieve comparability to identify causes. Thus, a representative sample may or may not include comparable exposed and unexposed members, and a purposive sample may or may not be representative of a particular population of interest. However, we separate these concepts to delineate the central concerns for each.

In the following sections, first we provide an overview of taking a representative sample of a population. Second, we provide an overview of three specific ways of sampling from a dynamic population to estimate measures of association for identification of causal effects.

How to Take a Representative Sample: The Basics

The most basic approach to taking a representative sample is to consider each member of the population as having an equal and independent probability of being selected into the sample. We can think of many events that are equally probable that we encounter in other areas of life, such as flipping a coin or rolling a dice. Assuming a fair coin, there is an equal probability that we will obtain a heads or a tails on a toss: 50% for each. Assuming a fair dice, there is an equal probability that we will roll each number, 1 through 6: the probability of each would be approximately 16.67%, or 1 in 6. Thus, to take a representative sample, in the simplest case, we first enumerate all potential members of the sample totaling the population size and assign each member a probability of being selected that is 1 over the population size. When the probability of being selected into the sample is approximately the same for each member of the population, and the selection of any particular member of the sample does not influence the selection of any other member (i.e., the probability of selection for each member is independent of any other member), we label the sample as a simple random sample. Although in lay contexts, random usually signifies something that is unpredictable or haphazard, in probability and statistics, random has a very specific definition. By a simple random sample, we mean that the probability of selection is approximately the same for each individual in the population, and the selection of each person is independent of the selection of other people.

As an example, we return to our hypothetical population of Farrlandia, and suppose we wish to take a simple random sample of the population at a single given time point. If the simple random sampling is successful (i.e., each person had an equal and independent probability of being selected), the sample should have the same basic characteristics as the population. The population noted in Figure 4.1 consists of 50 individuals, 25 of whom are exposed to

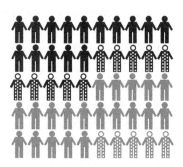

FIGURE 4.1 Population of Farrlandia consisting of 50 individuals.

a variable of interest (black), and 25 of whom are not (grey). We also indicate in the figure that some are dotted and some are not. These dots could represent another factor of interest, such as age, or cigarette smoking, or living in poverty or not. In the population, 15 individuals have dots. Taken together, the population has the following characteristics:

50% Exposed
30% Dotted

The goal of any random sampling technique is to collect a sample in such a way that approximately 50% are exposed and 30% are dotted.

We take a simple random sample of half of the population. Because it is a simple random sample, we would like each individual to have an equal probability of being selected, which would be 1/50 or 2%. To select individuals for the sample, one method would be to use a random number generator. Using any basic statistical software program, we can generate a series of numbers that lack any systematic pattern (i.e., are generated randomly). Because we want to select half of the population, we select people into the sample if the last digit of the random number generated for that individual is an even number (we could similarly decide that we are only going to take those with an odd number at the end). And, because we are randomly sampling, the individuals in Figure 4.2 should have the same distribution of sex, exposure, and dots as the population in Figure 4.1.

In our simple random sample of 25, we achieve close to the same distributions of black/gray and dots/no dots as in the population. We have 13 black individuals, representing 52% of the sample, and 8 dotted individuals, representing 32% of the sample. Thus, our simple random sample of the population is a good approximation of the distribution of color and dots as in the underlying population.

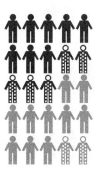

FIGURE 4.2 Random sampling using random number generator.

We provide an additional example of random sampling and the possibilities for getting it right versus wrong (Box 4.1) and provide an overview of one extension of the simple random sample (Box 4.2) in the online material that accompanies Chapter 4.

Quantifying Sampling Variability

Any time we take a sample from an underlying population, it is unlikely that the estimates that we generate will be exactly the same as the population parameters we would have calculated had we obtained information on the whole population. For instance, in our preceding example, taking a sample of 25 people from a population of 50, the distribution of color and dots was slightly higher than the underlying population. Consider the population of 20 people at high risk for diabetes, described in Figure 4.3. Of the 20 people, 8 are grey and 12 are black, indicating some kind of exposure; 10 of them have diabetes, indicated by Xs, and we are looking to estimate the proportion of the population with diabetes. Thus, the true population proportion is 50% (10/20). We want to take a sample of 5 people from this population of 20 people to estimate the population proportion of diabetes from a sample. Imagine

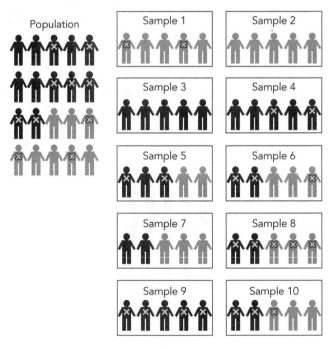

FIGURE 4.3 Variations in possible samples from a single population.

we took a random sample, measured diabetes, and took another random sample, measured diabetes among the 5 individuals in that sample, and then did this exercise again until we had thousands of random samples of 5 from this population of 20 people. In Figure 4.3, we show 10 possible samples of 5 people from the population of 20. In fact, there are 15,504 different groups of 5 that we could select from the group of 20 people. By chance, we might select all grey people. Also by chance, we might end up with a sample in which none of the individuals have diabetes, or one in which all of the individuals have diabetes. We can conceptualize all possible combinations of samples, some of which would render us reasonable estimates of the population proportion of diabetes and some of which would be way off.

What do we do in the face of this uncertainty? We can quantify this uncertainty and use it to provide numerical bounds that define a range of plausible values for the population parameter. There is a theorem that allows us to do this, the central limit theorem (CLT). Essentially, the CLT helps us understand three important points.

First, had we taken thousands of samples from our population of 20, the average proportion of diabetes across all of those samples would be identical to the true population proportion. Some samples would have had sample proportions of 100%, others would have had sample proportions of 0%, and still others would have had sample proportions between 0% and 100%, but the average of all of these sample proportions will be equal to the population proportion: 50%.

Second, the CLT tells us something about the variance (or spread) of those sample proportions across the distribution. Keeping with our hypothetical example of thousands of samples of size 5 people from our population of 20, we have an average of 50% and a range of 0% to 100%. The variability around the average can be quantified by

$$\sqrt{\frac{p(1-p)}{n}}$$

where p is the sample proportion and n is the sample size; we refer to this number as the *standard error*.

Third, provided a large sample size, the distribution of the thousands of sample proportions will be approximately normal (details on a normal distribution are given in the online material that accompanies this chapter), indicating that the shape of the distribution is symmetrical with a peak at the average sample proportion. How large is large? A typical rule of thumb is that samples should contain at least 30 individuals. Further, when examining binary categories of exposed and unexposed or diseased and nondiseased, there should be no group (e.g., exposed and diseased, unexposed and diseased, exposed and nondiseased, unexposed and nondiseased) smaller than 5. Note that these are rules of thumb and not mathematical axioms; thus, they should be followed generally rather than absolutely.

Given these three points, we can now put a bound around the sample proportion that quantifies our uncertainty due to sampling variability by estimating the standard error. As we see in the preceding formula for standard error, this measure of variability is determined by two principal factors—the proportion in the sample and the sample size. Sample size is central to quantifying uncertainly around our estimates. In the situation in which the population is 20 people, would we feel more confident in an estimate that comes from a sample of 4 people or a sample of 15? The sample of 15 is more likely to be representative of the underlying population than the sample of 4 because it contains more of the population. The larger the sample size, the smaller the amount of uncertainty we have in the sample estimate we have drawn about that population.

Why are we discussing this? The standard error will become critical in future chapters as we begin to put confidence intervals around population parameters and measures of association so that we can quantify the role of sampling variability in producing the sample estimates that we have obtained. For the moment, it is important to understand simply that the sample we draw from a population might be not representative of that population simply by chance; and because of this, we have to account for the uncertainty in the sample characteristics in some way. We do this in epidemiology by estimating standard errors.

How to Take a Purposive Sample: The Basics

As we noted in the beginning of this chapter, there are situations in which we may not want to take a representative sample of a population of interest using the simple random sample or another random sampling approach. This may be because we cannot enumerate all members of the population of interest to ensure that each member has an equal probability of being selected (e.g., there is no population register from which to draw the sample). Alternatively, we may not be interested in estimating a population parameter such as the proportion of individuals with breast cancer or the mean blood pressure. Instead, we may be interested in whether a certain factor has a causal effect on at least some people. In these cases, a representative sample is not required; rather, sampling such that those exposed to the hypothesized cause and those unexposed to the hypothesized cause are comparable is the primary design element of importance. An example that is often provided (Rothman, Gallacher, & Hatch, 2013) to demonstrate this point is research in animal models; we do not select mice systematically to be representative of all mice. Instead, we breed mice that are as similar to each other as possible aside from the one part of the experiment that we wish to manipulate.

When designing a study in which representativeness is not a concern, careful and complete eligibility criteria are of central importance (see Chapter 2). Because of the fluidity of eligibility for any particular study population, it is common in epidemiology to conceptualize study participants not in terms of actual people who are in the sample, but as the time that they contribute to the study while eligible. Thus, each person is re-conceptualized as a number—the number of days, months, or years that they are eligible for inclusion in the study sample. We detail how to operationalize this in the next chapter, focusing on the estimation of person time. In the following, we detail basic study designs that are employed to assess the health of samples that are collected in a purposive manner (although these designs can be used for representative samples as well).

Study Design: Representative and Purposive Samples

Whether we have a representative sample or a purposive sample, there are several fundamental options for designing a study that examines the health of a sample in a population. Principally, we can study the sample at a particular moment in time, follow it forward in time, or examine the retrospective exposure history of a sample. The decision will depend on the research question, the information about the sample that is needed, and logistical as well as practical considerations. As an example, it may be of interest for public health planning to know what proportion of individuals in the population has high blood pressure. We can capture this information at a single moment in time. If, on the other hand, we want to know how many new cases of high blood pressure we can expect over a 5-year period, we would need to follow individuals initially free of high blood pressure forward in time, counting cases as they arise.

What matters most in this endeavor is the timing of the sample selection in relation to the disease process of interest. Therefore, we need to understand the disease process we are interested in and use that to inform when we sample. There are three principal options:

> Option 1: Sample a group of individuals at a moment in time regardless of whether they have the disease or not, measuring disease and potential causes at the same time—in essence, we take a snapshot of the population;
> Option 2: Sample a group of individuals who are disease free, following them forward to count who gets the disease and who does not;
> Option 3: Sample a group of individuals based on health indicator status, with some having the health indicator and some not, examining this exposure history.

Each of these three options will have implications for how we analyze the data and draw inference, which we detail in future chapters. For now, it is important only to conceptualize that there are multiple points in time in the trajectory of a population at which the sample can be drawn.

We visualize these options using an example from Farrlandia. In Figure 4.4, we visually depict a population at four time points—these could represent any unit of time. For this example, we use years as our unit of time. We can see that people enter the population and others exit the population (either through death, emigration, or by no longer meeting the eligibility criteria). Some individuals have the disease at Year 1 (indicated by an X in the center), and some individuals develop the disease during the course of the 3 ensuing years.

Given the population of Farrlandia over these 4 years, we now review the three common options for taking a sample (either representative or purposive).

Option 1: Sample a group of individuals at a moment in time regardless of whether they are exposed or not, or have the disease or not, measuring disease and exposures simultaneously and not following forward—in essence we take a snapshot of the population.

Populations are often dynamic, constantly changing with time. Within the context of a dynamic population in which people are entering and exiting across time, how do we capture the health conditions that are a burden on the population? First, we choose a moment in time to look into that population, and we choose a sample. If we imagine a population with people constantly entering and exiting every single day, we just hit a hypothetical pause button and choose our sample at that time. Any study that simply hits the pause button and samples a population at a single moment in time, counting cases of disease and potential causes at that point in time, is termed a *cross-sectional*

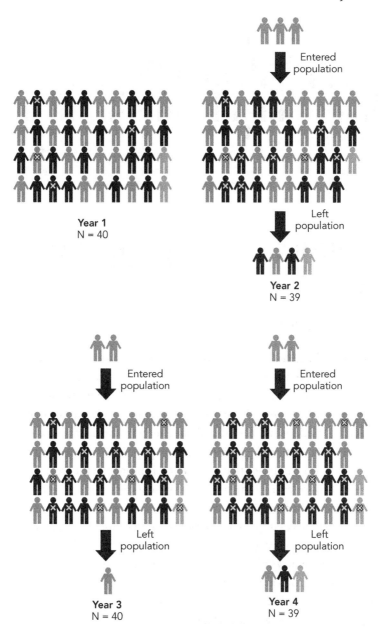

FIGURE 4.4 Population of Farrlandia over 4 years.

study; these studies are extensively used for surveillance of important health outcomes.

In Figure 4.5, we show an example of a cross-sectional sample at Year 3. Suppose we start our study in Year 3 of the 4-year depiction. Then the four people who left the population in Year 2 will not be included in our

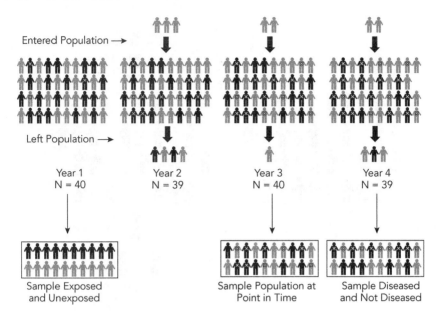

Entered Population →

Left Population →

Year 1	Year 2	Year 3	Year 4
N = 40	N = 39	N = 40	N = 39

Sample Exposed and Unexposed

Sample Population at Point in Time

Sample Diseased and Not Diseased

FIGURE 4.5 Taking different samples from a population.

assessment, and the two people who enter the population in Year 4 will not be included in our assessment. There is no definitively correct way to decide whether Year 1, Year 2, Year 3, or Year 4 will provide us with the most appropriate sample. Often the decision on when to start a study is more dependent on resources, funding, approvals, and time to get instruments ready to take into the field. Thus, thinking about dynamic populations and when to press pause and take the sample of that population is more of a theoretical exercise forcing us to consider how the study that we conduct is just one abstraction from a complex and dynamic process.

Note that when we sample a population at a single moment in time, we often cannot establish with certainty whether exposures occurred before the onset of disease, and we may miss cases of disease with short duration. Therefore, cross-sectional samples are often used to estimate population parameters such as the proportion of breast cancer or the mean symptoms of depression in the population of interest, rather than identifying causes of health indicators. Because of this, cross-sectional samples are more often representative samples than purposive samples. An example of a well-known representative cross-sectional sample is the National Health and Nutrition Examination Study (NHANES), conducted by the Centers for Disease Control and Prevention (http://www.cdc.gov/nchs/nhanes.htm). NHANES is conducted every 2 years to, among many goals, estimate the burden of various adverse health outcomes in the United States. NHANES is nationally representative, meaning that each 2-year sample is taken to represent the characteristics of all individuals living in households in the United States at that moment in time. Through the NHANES, we know what proportion of people in the United States have conditions such as cardiovascular disease, cancer, and many infectious diseases and also the proportion of people engaging in health behaviors of interest such as smoking and consuming high-fat foods. We do not need to follow individuals over time to estimate the current burden of disease in the United States—we need only a cross-section of the population at a single point in time.

Option 2: Sample a group of individuals who are disease free and following them forward to count who gets the disease and who does not.

We can also take a sample by focusing not on a particular time point but on whom to sample. We show an example of this sampling technique in Figure 4.5 at Year 1. We collect a sample of only those who are disease free. Using our sample of disease-free individuals, we can categorize individuals as exposed or unexposed. In Figure 4.5, exposure is noted by whether an individual is colored black or grey. We could collect a sample of 50% exposed and 50% unexposed (purposive sample) or allow the prevalence of exposure to represent the population-average exposure level (representative sample). Once collected, we follow this disease-free group forward in time and begin to count the cases of disease that arise. (In Chapters 5 and 6, we describe how to analyze this type of sample.) In epidemiology, studies that use this type of sampling are called cohort studies, prospective studies, or longitudinal studies.

Sampling a certain number of exposed and unexposed individuals (rather than a purely representative sample) may be of interest if the exposure is particularly rare. In the situation of a rare exposure, a representative sample would yield only a small number of exposed persons; collecting a purposive sample may be a more efficient study design. Second, we remind the reader that in the longitudinal study design we no longer conceptualize study participants as individuals but collections of time that are contributed to the study. Thus, if an individual is followed for 3 years, we would conceptualize this person as 3 person years rather than one person. Studies in which groups of individuals are followed forward in time are given several common names, depending on the discipline. In epidemiology, they are often referred to as *cohort studies,* but may also be termed *prospective* or *longitudinal studies.*

Option 3: Sample a group of individuals based on disease status, with some having the disease and some being disease free.

In Option 2 we described how we could collect a sample of all disease-free individuals, with a certain proportion exposed and a certain proportion unexposed. An alternative approach would be to sample a certain number of people who have the health indicator and a certain number who do not, and assess which group is more likely to be exposed. This is shown in Figure 4.5 at Year 4. Again, this can be done at any time point, but suppose we choose Year 4 to collect a group of individuals, half of whom have the disease and half of whom do not (see Year 4 in Figure 4.5). These types of studies are commonly done in hospitals, when a collection of patients with a certain disease or outcome are compared with respect to exposure to a group without the condition. Individuals with the disease and individuals without are typically purposefully sampled at a specific ratio. For example, we may collect one person without the disease for every person with the disease (1:1 sampling). It is also very common to select two people without the disease for every one with the disease (1:2 sampling). These types of studies are one form of a *case control study*.

The case control design is commonly used yet often misunderstood. In epidemiologic case control studies, a principal concern for validity is a well-defined population base of exposed and unexposed person times from which the cases and non-cases (controls) are drawn, even if such a population base has not been specifically enumerated (i.e., the population base can be hypothetical). Case control studies in epidemiology are conceptualized no differently from a study in which individuals are followed forward in time; the only difference is that we often collect the cases and non-cases at the end of some hypothetical follow-up period rather than then observing the cases arise over time from an underlying group of person times.

Figure 4.6 provides a visual description of a case control study within the context of an underlying population base. We begin with a cohort of 26 individuals who are initially free of the health indicator of interest and followed over a specified time period. Most population bases are of course much larger than 26 people, but we use this simple example as a heuristic. At the end of the time period, 10 individuals have developed the health indicator of interest, and 16 have not. In the case control design, we conceptualize taking a sample of the individuals who have the health indicator and a sample of those who do not have the health indicator. Suppose that we sample five cases, and two non-cases for every case as controls. Thus, we have a total sample of 15 individuals from our underlying base of 26 individuals, selected based on whether they have the health indicator or not (five cases, 10 controls).

In most case control studies (for exceptions, see Box 4.3 in the online material that accompanies this chapter), however, we do not have information on

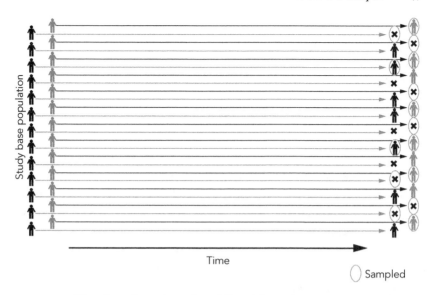

Time

◯ Sampled

FIGURE 4.6 Hypothetical population base followed forward over time, cases, and control sampled at the end of the follow-up period.

the underlying population base. For example, many case control studies are conducted within hospital or clinic settings. That is, we have access to cases of a health indicator, and then we need to select the appropriate control group for the case group. We may choose that control group from other individuals in the hospital, admitted for conditions other than the health indicator of interest, individuals from the community surrounding the hospital, friends or family members of the case, or another type of control. The principle concern in selecting this control group should be a group that is from the same population base that gave rise to the cases, even if such a population base has not been enumerated. That is, all of the cases should be eligible to have been in the control group had they not been cases, and all of the controls should have been eligible to be in the control group had they developed the health indicator of interest. Thus, the population base and subsequent sample is often hypothetical rather than literal.

Note that it is exceedingly rare to conduct a representative case control study. That is, we do not take a representative sample of all cases and a representative sample of all non-cases in a population. Nor do we need to. Rather, almost all case control studies employ purposive sampling, collected in an attempt to estimate whether the exposure of interest has a causal effect on the health indicator of interest. Further, note that although cases and controls sampled at the end of a hypothetical follow-up period is the most common conceptualization, case control studies can be conducted using other sampling techniques as well. We detail these additional sampling techniques in Box 4.3 of the online material that accompanies this chapter. Analytic and internal validity considerations for the case control design is discussed in future chapters.

Summary

In epidemiology we want to study populations—whole populations—but this is often infeasible. Thus, we take samples of dynamically moving populations. For some research questions, such as estimating the proportion of individuals with a certain health outcome, representative samples are necessary. In these situations we enumerate all individuals in the population and then randomly sample a certain number of them. When we have a random sample, the estimates that we obtain will likely be close to the population parameter of interest, and we use the standard error to put a bound around the variability in our sample that could be due to random chance in the sampling process. For other research questions, such as understanding whether pollution exposure causes lung cancer, representative samples are not necessary. We instead select people on the basis of exposure status or outcome status, and term these types of studies purposive samples.

Regardless of whether we collect a representative or purposive sample, we can collect our sample at different time points in the trajectory of a population and with different characteristics. We can take a snapshot sample of the population at a specific moment in time, measuring who happens to have the disease and who does not at that time. We can collect a sample ensuring that they are disease free, and then following them forward through time to see who gets the disease and who does not. We can also collect a sample based on disease status, collecting individuals who do and do not have the disease at a specific ratio. All of these methods for collecting samples are at the core different ways to look at a dynamic population to capture a piece of that population for the purposes of an epidemiologic study.

Reference

Rothman, K. J., Gallacher, J. E., & Hatch, E. E. (2013). Why representativeness should be avoided. *International Journal of Epidemiology*, *42*, 1012–1014.

5

Watching a Sample, Counting Cases

MOVING THROUGH OUR seven steps for epidemiologic studies, in Chapter 4 we addressed the third step: taking a sample. In this chapter, we begin to address Step 4. In Step 4, we examine whether there is the association between exposures and health indicators of interest. To test associations, we first need to assess the amount of the health indicator that occurs in both the exposed and unexposed group. Therefore, in this chapter, we review standard measures that are used to provide informative summaries of disease occurrence and frequency in our samples.

Before proceeding, we make special note of material that is available in the online material that accompanies this chapter. First, we focus throughout this textbook on basic measures of binary events in population health, that is, whether the health indicator is present or absent. We do this because these measures are foundational to understanding basic epidemiologic study design and analysis. However, a health indicator is often not measured as present versus absent; rather, it is measured in terms of gradations. Examples include blood pressure, cholesterol, BMI, birth weight, lung function, number of symptoms of depression or anxiety disorders, and many others. In these cases, we need to describe the data in terms of measures of centrality and spread of the data. We cover basic measures of centrality and spread (including means and variances, median and mode) in Box 5.1 of the online material that accompanies Chapter 5. Second, we note that in infectious disease epidemiology there are additional measures of occurrence that are important to consider. We provide an overview of basic reproductive rate, net reproductive rate, and herd immunity in Box 5.2 of the online material that accompanies Chapter 5.

Counts

Perhaps the most basic summary measure of disease in a population or sample is a simple count of the number of cases of the health indicator of interest that occur. Counts of cases provide a measure of the absolute burden of disease. However, they are limited in their utility.

Suppose we would like to estimate the burden of tuberculosis in New York City. In many locations, tuberculosis is a reportable condition, meaning that any health professional that diagnoses a case of tuberculosis must report it to the New York State Department of Health so that control measures can be taken if the number of cases is above what would be expected. In 2011, there were 689 reported new cases of tuberculosis in New York (New York State Department of Health, 2011). This alone gives us some information on the burden of disease in the population. Yet there are two problems with this measure for determining the burden of tuberculosis in New York.

First, what if we knew nothing about the total population size of New York? A case count of 689 is very different in terms of the population burden if the population size is 100,000 people versus 10,000,000 people. Given known information about the estimated size of the population, we can now estimate measures that tell us about the proportion of people in New York that are affected by tuberculosis.

Second, those who already have tuberculosis are not at risk for developing a new onset of tuberculosis. It is important for public health to be able to estimate the population at risk; to do that, we need to know something about the existing cases of tuberculosis in New York. We know that 689 people in New York were diagnosed in 2011, but how many were diagnosed in 2010—and 2009? Knowing the proportion of new cases divided by the number of individuals who are at risk for developing tuberculosis provides additional information about the distribution of the disease in the population.

The two measures of disease that help us overcome these challenges are called prevalence and risk. Prevalence is a measure of the total burden of tuberculosis overall in the population. Prevalence tells us the proportion of cases among the total population at any given time. A measure of new cases of disease among the population at risk is termed the risk. In this chapter we discuss these measures in more detail.

Prevalence

Prevalence tells us about the total burden of disease at any given time. To determine the overall burden, we estimate the proportion of people who have the disease (existing cases plus new cases) over the total population for a given time period:

$$\text{Prevalence over time } t \ = \ \frac{\text{Number with the health indicator of interest}}{\text{Total population size}}$$

Figure 5.1 shows a sample of 30 individuals across 3 years from our fictional population of Farrlandia. In Year 1, 5 individuals developed the health indicator of interest. In Year 2, an additional 7 people developed the health indicator of interest. Because this hypothetical health indicator is not curable, the 5 individuals who developed the health indicator in Year 1 still have the health indicator in Year 2. In Year 3, an additional 4 individuals developed the health indicator of interest.

What is the prevalence of disease in Year 2? We need a numerator, a denominator, and a time period of interest. We have 5 cases of disease from Year 1 who still have the disease and 7 new cases in Year 2. Therefore, we have 12 existing cases in the numerator. The denominator is the total sample size,

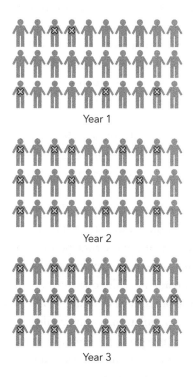

FIGURE 5.1 Disease occurrence in a sample of Farrlandia over time.

that is, 30 individuals. Thus, the prevalence of disease is 12/30 = 0.40, or 40% in Year 2. What is the prevalence of disease in Year 3? Now we add the 5 people from Year 1, plus the 7 people from Year 2, and the 4 people in Year 3 to get a total of 16 in the numerator. The denominator is still the total sample size of 30. The prevalence of disease in Year 3 is 16/30 = 0.533, or 53.3%, which means that 53.3% of the sample has the disease in Year 3. We note that the time period should be specified as precisely as possible. When we say in Year 3, we mean over the duration of Year 3. We could also, however, specify prevalence on June 5 in Year 3, and that prevalence may well be different than the prevalence on December 14. Specifying such time point prevalence depends on having accurate counts for the numerator and denominator at particular moments in time.

Risk

Risks are perhaps the most widely used tools in epidemiology. *Risk* is a proportion indicating the number of new cases divided by the number of individuals in the sample at risk of becoming a case. The broad utility of risk measures has led them to be given many names by different epidemiology books over time. We use the term *risk* throughout the book, but note other equally common terms, including "incidence" or, less commonly, "incidence proportion." As in the case of prevalence, to estimate this measure we need a numerator, a denominator, and a time period of interest.

$$\text{Risk over time } t = \frac{\text{Number who develop the health indicator of interest}}{\substack{\text{Total number at risk of developing} \\ \text{the health indicator of interest}}}$$

The numerator is the number of new cases that were diagnosed in the time period of interest. The denominator is the total size of the population at risk of developing the outcome during the time period of interest. Those who are at risk are the individuals who could conceivably develop the outcome. This excludes people who already have the outcome as well as people who could not possibly develop the outcome. For example, if we wanted to estimate the risk of uterine cancer in a population, whom would we include in the denominator? First, we would remove from the denominator those who already have uterine cancer at the beginning of the time period in which we are estimating new cases. We would also need to remove men, as they cannot conceivably develop the outcome. Further, we would want to remove women who have had a hysterectomy, as they also cannot develop uterine cancer. Similarly, if we want to estimate the risk of prostate cancer, we would remove women from the denominator, as they do not have a prostate.

We go back to Figure 5.1.

What is the risk of disease in the sample of Farrlandia in Year 2?

We need three pieces of information to estimate risk: the number of new cases (numerator), the population at risk (denominator), and a time period of interest. The time period of interest is Year 2. The numerator would be 7 because 7 people developed the disease in Year 2. What is the denominator? Because 5 people already had the disease, we would not want to count them; thus, 25 people were at risk of developing the disease in Year 2. The risk is thus 7/25, or 0.28, or 28% in Year 2. We should always include the time period of interest in our reporting of risk. To understand why, consider if we wanted to know the risk across both Years 2 and 3? In the numerator, we add the number of people who develop the disease across these 2 years: 7 in Year 2, and 4 in Year 3 for a total of 11. Our denominator is still 25 individuals, as 25 were at risk of developing disease at the beginning of Year 2, when we begin counting. Thus, the 2-year risk is 11/25 = 0.44, or 44% in Years 2 and 3. The measure that we calculate is dependent on the time period that we are examining; we note that the 1-year risk in Year 2 is 28% and the 2-year risk across Years 2 and 3 is 44%.

Risk Versus Prevalence: The Bathtub Analogy

Figure 5.2 shows the classic bathtub example, which illustrates the relation between prevalence and risk. The basin of the bathtub holds all of the individuals with a health indicator of interest. Water from the spout can be thought of as the introduction of new cases in the population (risk). High risk of the health indicator is equivalent to a strong flow from the spout. The drain represents exit from the population of individuals with the health indicator, either through death or recovery.

We consider a few examples within the context of the bathtub analogy to understand the relation between risk and prevalence over time.

High Risk, Steady Prevalence

If a health indicator has a high risk (many new cases) over time and a steady prevalence over time that is approximately equal to the risk, this is equivalent to a strong flow of water coming into the bathtub but with a very wide drain. Very little water can accumulate in the bathtub basin. Consider an infectious

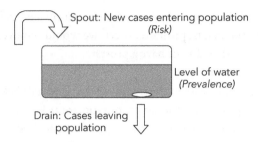

FIGURE 5.2 Understanding risk and prevalence: the bathtub example.

disease with a very short duration, or one that has a very high case fatality (i.e., a high proportion of cases die from the illness). Even if the risk of such a disease is high, the prevalence will remain steady and approximately equivalent to risk because no water is accumulating in the basin. In other words, the water is leaving through the drain (either from recovery or death) as quickly as it is coming in.

Low Risk, High Prevalence

Health indicators with long duration such as arthritis, diabetes, Crohn's disease, and other chronic illnesses may have a constant overall risk but an increasing prevalence over time. If very little water is leaving the bathtub (i.e., few individuals recover from the disease but the duration of the disease is very long), then prevalence will become relatively high over time even if risk is relatively low. We can conceptualize this as the water accumulating in the basin.

The Impact of New Treatments That Affect Duration

Given this understanding of risk and prevalence, we can now conceptualize how new treatments may affect risk and prevalence differently. Consider the example of antiretroviral therapy (ART) for management of HIV symptoms. Prior to the introduction of ART medications, duration of illness with HIV was on average relatively short, with a rapid progression to AIDS and eventual death from the disease (Murphy et al., 2001). ART allowed HIV-positive individuals to live much longer lives, but it did not cure the disease. Thus, duration increased substantially. We can consider this as the closing of the bathtub drain. Once ART was introduced, even if risk is affected at all, we expect an increasing prevalence of the disease over time as individuals lived longer lives with the disease. This is illustrated in Figure 5.3.

The increase in prevalence given an increase in duration of disease can occur independently of risk. That is, for noninfectious diseases, an increase in

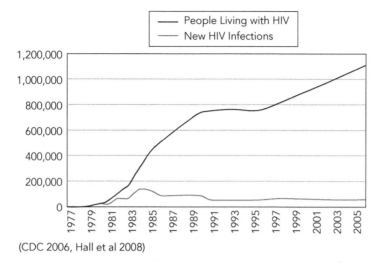

(CDC 2006, Hall et al 2008)

FIGURE 5.3 Estimated number of new HIV infections and persons living with HIV, 1977–2006.

Adapted from "HIV prevalence estimates—United States, 2006," by Centers for Disease Control and Prevention (CDC), 2008, *Morbidity and Mortality Weekly Report*, *57*, p. 1074; and "Estimation of HIV incidence in the United States," By H. I. Hall, R. Song, P. Rhodes, J. Prejean, Q. An, L. M. Lee, . . . HIV Incidence Surveillance Group, 2008, *Journal of the American Medical Association*, *300*, p. 520–529.

duration of disease will increase the prevalence without affecting risk in any way. For HIV/AIDS, risk may also be affected because a greater proportion of people living longer with HIV/AIDS could translate to an increased number of new cases assuming that increasing duration also increases the length of time in which someone would be able to transmit the disease to others.

Summary

In all of the preceding examples, the key to the relation between risk and prevalence in a particular population is the average duration of the disease. Over time, risk and prevalence will be approximately equal when the duration of disease is very short. Prevalence will be higher than overall risk across the same time period when duration of the disease is very long.

Incidence Rates

The measure of risk that we described earlier in the chapter is most accurate when the distribution of case development across the time period of interest is relatively even, and each individual is observed at every measurement time point from the beginning of the study to the end. Neither of these may hold for a given health indicator. We motivate the potential problems in using risks with two examples.

Consider two studies in which the number of new cases of a particular disease is measured over 12 months. Both follow 100,000 individuals at risk for developing the disease; and in both studies, 120 individuals develop the disease over the 12 months. In the first study, there were 10 new cases every month. In the second study, all 120 individuals developed the disease in the first month. These studies would report the same risk (120/100,000), but we might want to capture the different dynamics of the disease occurrence over time between these two studies.

We consider a second example. Suppose we are interested in the relation between alcohol consumption and liver cirrhosis. We collect a sample of 10 individuals who are heavy drinkers (we call these people exposed, marked in black) and 10 individuals who are not heavy drinkers (we call these people unexposed, marked in grey). None of these individuals have liver cirrhosis. We then follow these individuals forward in time, with an interest in determining which individuals develop liver cirrhosis. Every 10 years we bring the sample back to see who has developed the outcome—in this case, who has cirrhosis. Figure 5.4 shows our ideal scenario. We are able to track information on all 20 of our individuals. At Time 2, 3 have cirrhosis (2 exposed and 1 unexposed). At Time 3, an additional 3 people have cirrhosis for a total of 6 cases (4 exposed and 2 unexposed). At Time 4, an additional 7 people have cirrhosis (4 exposed and 3 unexposed.) By the last time point of follow-up, we have a total of 13 cases: 8 among the exposed and 5 among the unexposed.

In Chapter 6, we detail how we would estimate associations between exposure and outcome in this sample; but for the moment, we focus on overall cirrhosis regardless of heavy drinking status. Out of our original sample of 20 people, 13 have cirrhosis over 40 years. Thus, the cirrhosis risk in our sample is 65%.

But what if we did not follow all of the people the whole time? Some people could drop out of our study, perhaps by moving to a different location and not providing us with follow-up information. In Figure 5.5, we provide such an example. Now, at Time 2, we have one person drop out, denoted by a dotted box. We know that this person is unexposed, but we do not know whether she developed cirrhosis. At Time 3, two more people drop out for a total of three lost individuals. Finally at Time 4, an additional two people drop out, for a total of five lost individuals.

How do we calculate cirrhosis risk in our sample, given these five dropouts?

One way would be to estimate cirrhosis risk among just those who finished the study. Out of the 15 people who finished the study, we know that

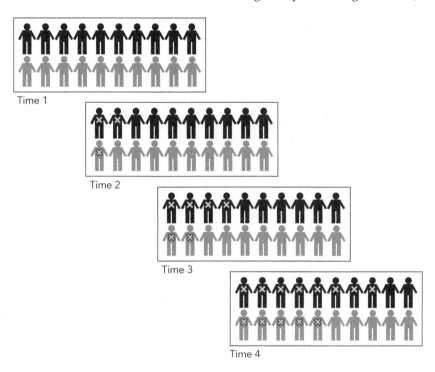

FIGURE 5.4 Disease risk over time by population exposure.

9 developed cirrhosis. We could estimate the risk of cirrhosis as 9/15 or 60%. This would underestimate the true risk of 65%. Note that the true risk is unknowable in our study with loss to follow-up because we do not have cirrhosis information on those lost.

Another option would be to estimate cirrhosis risk assuming that all of those who were lost did not develop cirrhosis. We know that 9 people developed cirrhosis out of the original 20, thus the risk is 9 out of 20 or 45%. This underestimates the true risk even more. A final option would be to assume that all of those who dropped out of the study developed cirrhosis. Then we would have a risk of cirrhosis of 14 out of 20 or 70%, which is an overestimate of the true risk of 65%.

There is one more option, which is to estimate an incidence rate. Incidence rates are very commonly used in epidemiology, especially in cohort studies (i.e., those in which we begin with a sample of people without disease and follow them forward in time) in which some people in the sample are lost over time.

To estimate an incidence rate for the time frame of the study, we need to know how much total time each person contributed to the study follow-up before they either developed the outcome or dropped out. To figure this out

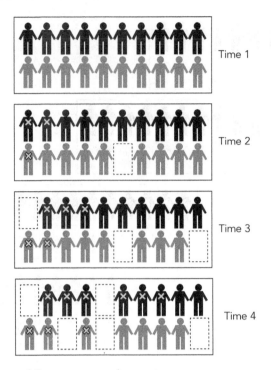

Time 1

Time 2

Time 3

Time 4

FIGURE 5.5 Loss to follow-up in a sample over time.

for the people in our study, consider the following example. We collect a group of 20 women in Farrlandia who are free of breast cancer. We follow them for 40 years, assessing every 10 years whether they develop breast cancer. Some women drop out of the study and some women die of non-breast cancer causes before the study is over. Our data are shown in Figure 5.6.

Person 2 stayed in the study for all four follow-ups and never developed breast cancer. Thus, this person contributed 40 years of disease-free time to the study. All individuals who stayed in the study for the whole period and never developed the outcome will contribute 40 years of disease-free time to the study. We have six of these individuals in the study.

Now we consider those who developed the outcome. We see that Person 19 already had breast cancer at the first follow-up. Ideally, we would like to know the exact minute when that individual developed the disease. Then we would know exactly how much time the individual was at risk before developing the outcome. It is almost impossible to know exactly when someone develops a disease, however, so we use an estimate.

We do not know exactly when this person developed breast cancer over the 10 years from the start of the study to the first follow-up; we assume that

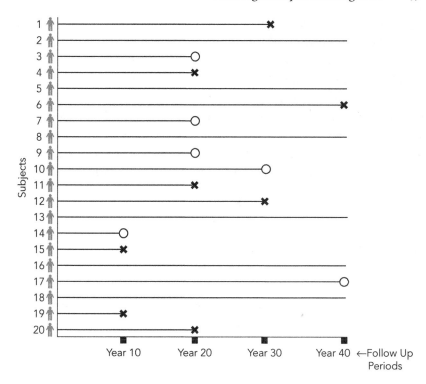

FIGURE 5.6 Understanding person years.

they developed the disease at the midpoint between the baseline and first follow-up (5 years). This person will no longer contribute any time to the study because they have the outcome of interest. Person 11 developed breast cancer by the second follow-up. We know that she was disease-free for the first 10 years of the study, and developed breast cancer somewhere in between the first and second follow-up. Thus, we add 5 additional years of disease-free time for Person 15 as the midpoint of the time between the first and second follow-up for a total of 15 years of disease-free time in the study. We calculate this same measure for each person in the study.

Finally, we discuss those individuals lost to follow-up. Person 3 was lost at the second follow-up. This person then contributed 10 years, because we knew that they were disease-free at baseline and at the first follow-up, but we have no information on them after that point. Person 10 was lost at the third follow-up. Thus, we know that this person was disease-free between baseline and the first follow-up, as well as between the first follow-up and second follow-up. Thus, this person contributed 20 years to the study in which we knew she was disease-free. We can estimate a similar measure of the number of disease-free years for all other individuals lost to follow-up. Our final calculations look like the data in Table 5.1.

The calculation of disease-free time for each individual is the person time. Recall from Chapter 4 that when we follow individuals over time, we no longer view them as a collection of people but rather as a collection of times. Calculating person time is a way to quantify this collection of times. Armed with information about person time, we can now calculate an incidence rate by dividing the number of new cases (in our final sample at the fourth follow-up, we have eight cases) by the total amount of person time contributed by all individuals in the sample:

$$\frac{8}{460} = .017$$

On average, our sample developed breast cancer at a rate of 17 new cases per 1,000 person years.

Table 5.1 Person Time and Disease Status Among 20 Subjects Followed for 40 Years

Subject	Years Contributed	Developed Disease? (0 no/1 yes)
1	25	1
2	40	0
3	10	0
4	15	1
5	40	0
6	35	1
7	10	0
8	40	0
9	10	0
10	20	0
11	15	1
12	25	1
13	40	0
14	0	0
15	5	1
16	40	0
17	30	0
18	40	0
19	5	1
20	15	1

The incidence rate can be interpreted as the number of expected cases in every set of 1,000 person years. That is, if we were to observe 1,000 people for 1 year, we would expect 17 cases. If we were to observe 500 people for 2 years, we would still expect 17 cases. The assumption underlying this is that the incidence rate is constant over time; thus, for every year in which 1,000 person years are observed, an additional 17 cases will be expected. Given this assumption, the incidence rate tells us the average number of cases per specified set of person time.

In additional to estimating disease occurrence and frequency, risk, rate, and prevalence, measures can be used to inform a wide range of other measures of disability and morbidity related to disease and health. Disability is typically conceptualized in a health context as a broad term encompassing any type of impairment or reduced functioning in daily life and may be due to symptoms or diseases. Disabilities are context dependent, as the reduction in functioning depends on environmental conditions and barriers. In Box 5.3 of the online material that accompanies Chapter 5, we review a commonly used measure of disability in populations—disability adjusted life years (DALYs).

Rate Versus Proportion: What Is the Difference?

It is worth pausing for a moment to reinforce the differences between a rate and a proportion. When we refer to the risk of a health indicator, we refer to the proportion of new cases in the population at risk. A proportion can range from 0 to 100, and the numerator is part of the denominator. An incidence rate, on the other hand, can range from 0 to infinity; and the numerator is the number of cases, whereas the denominator is the person time at risk. A rate can be conceptualized as a measure of speed. We use rates in our daily lives when we measure the speed at which we are driving in miles per hour; incidence rates can be conceptualized as the speed at which disease is occurring in cases per person year. When we have complete follow-up of a sample or a population, the rate can approximate the proportion of disease or the risk. Consider the following example. We have 10 people who are disease-free at the start of follow-up, each followed for 1 year; 3 of these individuals develop the disease. All individuals are followed for the entirety of the study period. The risk of disease will be 3 out of 10, or 0.30. Assuming these individuals were assessed for the development the disease just as the year was ending, the rate would be 3 per 10 person years or 0.30. If we apply the algorithm specified previously to take the midpoint of the time interval

---

BOX 5.1

Risk, Incidence, and Incidence Rate

Because measures of incidence are central to epidemiologic investigation, the term *incidence* can be used in various contexts, and the concept that we refer to as "incidence" can go by different terms. We clarify this here:

Incidence: The incidence refers to the number of new cases divided by the population at risk. It is also called the incidence proportion, or the risk.

Finally, in infectious disease settings, the term *attack rate* is often used to describe the number of cases of an infectious disease over the population at risk. Thus, it is not technically a rate and is synonymous with risk, incidence, and incidence proportion:

Incidence rate: The incidence rate refers to the number of new cases divided by the person time at risk contributed by members of the study.

Throughout this book, we use the term *risk* to describe the incidence or incidence proportion. When we refer to incidence rate, we specifically refer to a measure in which the denominator is the person time at risk contributed by members of the study.

---

for those who developed the disease as those individual's person times, we would have the following:

7   people were followed and did not develop the disease—1 person year for each totaling 7 person years.
3   people developed the disease—we assign each of them 0.5 person years for the midpoint of the time interval for a total of 1.5 person years.

Thus, the incidence rate would be 3 per 8.5 person years, or 0.35.

Rates reflect the disease incidence under the circumstance of incomplete follow-up more accurately than risks because they maximize the information from each participant. We summarize and clarify the terminology around incidence and incidence rate in Box 5.1 in this chapter.

Conditional Risks: The Start of Examining Association

In Chapter 6, we formally discuss how to use these measures of disease occurrence to estimate associations between exposures and health indicators of interest. Here we note that once we have measures of disease occurrence, we can condition those measures on other factors of interest: that is, calculate them in different subgroups. For simplicity we discuss risks, but the same logic can be applied to rates, means, medians, and modes.

As an example, suppose we are interested in whether condom use influences risk of trichomoniasis among sexually active adolescents. We obtain a sample of 20 adolescents in the population of Farrlandia and follow them for 1 year; for this example, we assume that there was no loss to follow-up. Thus, estimates of risk should sufficiently capture the infection occurrence in our sample. In Figure 5.4, we determined that the overall risk of trichomoniasis in our sample was 65%. Because we hypothesize that condom use will protect adolescents from the development of trichomoniasis, we label the exposed as non-condom users and the unexposed as condom users.

To estimate whether condom users have a different risk of trichomoniasis compared with non-condom users, we can use a measure of the conditional risk. We condition the estimation on a certain variable and estimate risk only among those with the variable. In this case, we want to know the risk of trichomoniasis conditional on being a condom user versus the risk of trichomoniasis conditional on not being a condom user.

As a means of organizing the information taking into account now two factors, condom use and trichomoniasis, we create a 2 × 2 table as shown in Figure 5.7.

In Figure 5.8 we cross-classify those who use condoms with those who have trichomoniasis or not. We now fill in the cells of that 2 × 2 table counting the number of individuals who were both exposed (did not use condoms) and developed trichomoniasis, and those who were unexposed (used condoms) and developed trichomoniasis. Note that we also include the total number of

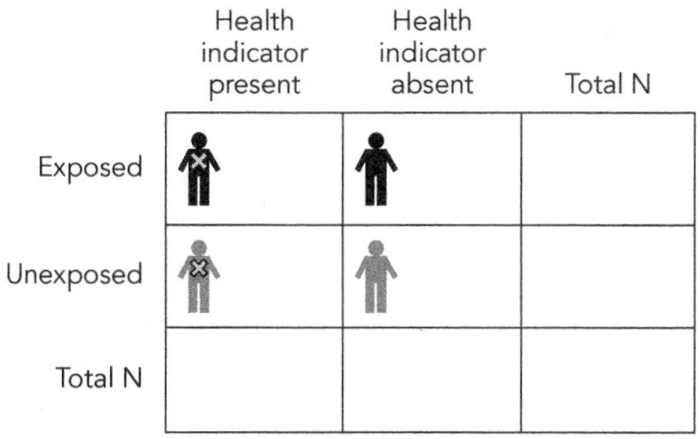

FIGURE 5.7 A 2 × 2 table showing exposure status in each row and disease status in each column.

	Health indicator present	Health indicator absent	Total N
Exposed	8	2	10
Unexposed	5	5	10
Total N	13	7	20

FIGURE 5.8 Association between condom use and trichomoniasis.

exposed and unexposed, health indicator present and health indicator absent, in this table. Thus, it technically becomes 3 × 3 rather than 2 × 2. However, the terminology "2 × 2 table" is canonical in epidemiology and refers to the separation of exposure and health indicator status; thus, we retain the terminology 2 × 2 table throughout this text.

We see here that we have 8 non-condom users with trichomoniasis, 2 non-condom users without trichomoniasis, 5 condom users with trichomoniasis, and 5 condom users without trichomoniasis.

Before estimating the conditional risks, notice what we call the *marginal numbers*. Marginal numbers are those that are at the margins of the 2 × 2 table. Combining both exposed and unexposed with trichomoniasis, we see that there are 13 overall adolescents with trichomoniasis in the sample of 20 people. The overall risk in the sample is thus 13/20 = 65%.

Next, we condition on the exposure status to estimate the risk of trichomoniasis among those exposed (non-condom users) and those unexposed (condom users). The denominator will now change from the total sample to only those with the condition of interest.

Under the condition of exposure (non-condom use), we have 8/10 with trichomoniasis.

Under the condition of not being exposed (condom use), we have 5/10 with trichomoniasis.

Thus, it appears that the risk of trichomoniasis (80%) seems to be higher in the exposed than in the unexposed (50%). Although 80% appears to be higher than 50%, remember that we took a sample of the population to estimate these risks. Through variability in the sampling process, we could have arrived at these seemingly different risks just by chance alone. Thus we need additional tools to evaluate these differences in risk.

Confidence Intervals for Rates and Proportions

The measures that we have described can be estimated within a sample of a population or computed from an entire population. If we estimate measures of disease occurrence within a sample, we need to account for sampling variability. As we described in Chapter 4, sampling variability refers to the fact that if we take a random sample of a population, the estimate that we get may not be the same as we would have gotten if we had information on the whole population or from a different sample of that population. We discussed the idea of a thought experiment: we have a population, and we take thousands of different random samples of that population. We then estimate the risk of a health indicator in each of these thousands of samples. The average of all of those thousands of risk estimates in the sample will be the true underlying risk in the population, and the variability around that population risk can be estimated with the standard error. In the following, we provide an overview of standard error estimation and the resulting construction and meaning of a confidence interval for two measures: proportions and rates. We provide an overview of standard error calculation for means in Box 5.4 of the online material that accompanies Chapter 5. Standard errors and confidence intervals for other measures of occurrence such as medians and modes become more complicated; thus, for the introductory student we recommend mastering the proportions, rates, and means before moving to more complex standard error estimates.

The standard error for a proportion is calculated as follows:

$$SE = \sqrt{\frac{p(1-p)}{n}},$$

where p is the sample proportion and n is the sample size. Proportions we have discussed in this chapter include prevalence and risk.

The standard error for a rate is calculated as follows:

$$SE = \sqrt{\frac{d}{PY^2}},$$

where d is the number of people with the outcome and PY is the total amount of person time in the study.

Now that we have a standard error for each of the estimates, we can then provide confidence intervals around these estimates. The confidence interval is a range of estimates for the population that are relatively consistent with the data given sampling variability. A standard in the epidemiologic literature is 95% confidence intervals, although in some circumstances we may wish to be more or less confident depending on the nature of the research question. For now, we proceed assuming that we would like to be 95% confident about our study estimates.

To understand the confidence interval, we return to our thought experiment. If we took thousands of random samples of the same size from the population, the 95% confidence interval technically tells us that that the true population value would be included in 95% of the resulting confidence intervals in those thousands of studies. Whether the true population value is in our particular confidence interval from our particular sample is unknown. But, the confidence interval gives us an indication of the range of values for the true population parameter that would generally be consistent with our data. For example, suppose that we take a sample of size 50 from the population of Farrlandia and estimate the proportion of individuals with hip fractures. Our sample statistic is 12%, indicating that 12% of our sample has a hip fracture. Without detailing the estimation of the confidence interval, suppose that our 95% confidence interval is from 10 to 14. This indicates that a reasonable range of values for the prevalence of hip fracture that would be consistent with our data is the range from 10% to 14%.

Confidence intervals thus provide a range of values around the sample estimate that indicates how confident we are in how well our study estimate reflects the true underlying population estimate. The confidence interval will become wider as the sample size becomes smaller because the smaller the sample size, the more likely we are to get a sample that does not reflect the true underlying population proportion or mean.

Next, we need to understand why the range of a 95% confidence interval would be from 10% to 14% in our hypothetical example. We have drawn thousands of random samples from the population and estimated the prevalence of hip fractures in each of those samples. If we were to plot prevalence from these thousands of samples by the number of occurrences of each prevalence estimate, we may find something like what is shown in Figure 5.9.

We know from the CLT (Chapter 4) that the average of those many thousands of samples will be the true population prevalence. We can also say something about the proportion of the sample's prevalence that will be near the population prevalence. As we describe in Box 5.5 of the online material that accompanies this chapter, about 68% of the prevalence that we estimate across those many thousands of samples will fall within 1 standard error of the population prevalence, and 95% will fall within approximately 2 standard errors

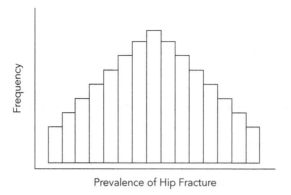

Prevalence of Hip Fracture

FIGURE 5.9 Hypothetical distribution of hip fracture prevalence in thousands of samples of size 50 drawn from the population of Farrlandia.

(e.g., the sample prevalence will be outside that range—about 2 standard errors above and 2 standard errors below—5% of the time). However, because we do not know the true underlying population prevalence, we use our sample estimate as our best guess about what the true population proportion is. Thus, when we estimate the 95% confidence interval around the sample prevalence, we estimate the range of values that we estimate to be approximately 2 standard errors above or below the true population prevalence if we took thousands of random samples of the same size from the same population.

In summary, we use the sample estimate of the prevalence, risk, and incidence rate as our best guess of the corresponding population parameter. We estimate the standard error for that sample estimate and calculate the range of values that is above or below about 2 standard errors of the sample estimate. This forms our 95% confidence intervals, which tells us the range of values and gives a measure of the range of plausible values for the population parameter of interest.

Here is the 95% confidence interval for a proportion:

$$p \pm 1.96(SE),$$

where p is the sample proportion; 1.96 is an approximation of 2 because we want approximately 2 standard errors above or below (see Box 5.5 in the online material that accompanies Chapter 5 for an explanation of the z distribution and why we use 1.96); and SE is the standard error for the proportion.

Here is the 95% confidence interval for a rate:

$$r \pm 1.96(SE),$$

where r is the sample incidence rate, and SE is the standard error of the rate.

Note that being 95% confident does not mean that there is a 95% chance that the true population parameter is in the interval. The only thing we know is that if we were to repeat the process of taking different samples over and over again, 95% of the intervals that we construct from those samples will contain the true population parameter—but 5% will not. In any particular sample, however, the confidence interval either contains the true population parameter or it does not. Whether our particular confidence interval contains the true population parameter we will never know with full certainty.

We make one final note regarding sample size. Remember from Chapter 4 that for the CLT to hold, we need the sample size to be large enough; and as a rule of thumb, we use sample sizes of at least 30 and all exposure/disease categories having at least 5 individuals. Thus, these confidence intervals provide reliable bounds accounting for sampling variability only to the extent that we have met the assumptions of the CLT and have large enough sample sizes.

Summary

In epidemiology, there are a number of measures that are useful to characterize the overall occurrence and frequency of disease. Cardinal measures include risk (also known as incidence, incidence proportion, and attack rate), prevalence, and incidence rate. Mean, variance, median, and mode are also important measures of occurrence in epidemiologic samples, which we cover in the online material that accompanies this chapter. Each of these measures has different properties and different circumstances in which they would be appropriate. Risk is appropriate when there is little loss to follow-up in the sample and relatively uniform distribution of cases across the time period of interest; otherwise, an incidence rate is preferable. The prevalence of disease is a function of the disease risk and duration. If duration of disease is increased, prevalence will increase, even if risk does not change or even if it decreases. When we take a sample of a population to estimate a measure of disease occurrence, it is important to provide a standard error or a confidence interval around our estimate to provide information about the precision of the estimate.

References

Centers for Disease Control and Prevention (CDC). (2008). HIV prevalence estimates—United States, 2006. *Morbidity and Mortality Weekly Report, 57*, 1073–1076.

Hall, H. I., Song, R., Rhodes P., Prejean, J., An, Q., Lee, L. M., . . . HIV Incidence Surveillance Group. (2008). Estimation of HIV incidence in the United States. *Journal of the American Medical Association, 300,* 520–529.

Murphy, E. L., Collier, A. C., Kalish, L. A., Assmann, S. F., Para, M. F., Flanigan, T. P., . . . Viral Activation Transfusion Study Investigators. (2001). Highly active antiretroviral therapy decreases mortality and morbidity in patients with advanced HIV disease. *Annals of Internal Medicine, 135,* 17–26.

New York State Department of Health, Bureau of Tuberculosis Control. (2011). *Tuberculosis in New York State—2011 annual statistical report.* Retrieved from http://www.health.ny.gov/statistics/diseases/communicable/tuberculosis/docs/2011_annual_report.pdf

6

Are Exposures Associated With Health Indicators?

STEP 3 IN our seven-step guide to conducting epidemiologic studies is estimating measures of association between exposures and health indicators of interest. In the previous chapter, we covered how to estimate measures of disease occurrence and frequency such prevalence, risks, and rates; in our online material we covered means, medians, and modes. Now that we understand how to quantify the occurrence of disease, we can now move to comparing the occurrence of health indicators between two groups, thus estimating measures of association. Note that for this chapter, we focus on measures of association for binary outcomes rather than those that are graded or continuous. We do this because binary health indicators (e.g., presence or absence of disease) form the foundational bedrock of epidemiologic studies. Therefore, mastery of these basic measures of association for binary measures is essential for the introductory student.

Introduction

In Chapter 5, we introduced how we can assess measures of disease occurrence and frequency conditionally on exposures. For example, we may be interested in the incidence of disease among those exposed and the incidence of disease among those unexposed. Once we have those two measures, we need tools to compare them to decide whether the overall incidence is higher among one group than another.

One way to compare two measures is simple visual examination. For example, suppose we conduct a study in Farrlandia in which 10,000 people free of heart disease are followed for 5 years; 3,000 of these individuals are smokers, and of these, 410 develop heart disease. The remaining 7,000 are nonsmokers

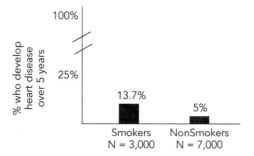

We study 10,000 people in the population of Farrlandia, 3,000 of whom are smokers. Among smokers, we can see that there is a higher percentage of individuals who develop heart disease than among nonsmokers. But for an epidemiologic study it is important to quantify this difference and provide an estimate of the strength of the difference between smokers and nonsmokers in terms of heart disease risk.

FIGURE 6.1   Incidence proportion of heart disease among 3,000 smokers and 7,000 nonsmokers in Farrlandia, observed over 5 years.

and of these, 350 develop heart disease. We assume that there is no loss to follow-up and no one quits smoking or starts smoking during the study time period.

In this scenario, the best measure of disease occurrence would be the risk (which, as we mentioned in Chapter 5, is also called the incidence). In Figure 6.1, we see that the risk of disease among the exposed (smokers) is

$$\frac{410}{3000} = 0.14,$$

The risk of disease among the nonsmokers is

$$\frac{350}{7000} = 0.05,$$

Clearly we can see that 14% is larger than 5%. But how do we quantify how much larger 14% is compared with 5%? How do we know if the difference between these two percentages is meaningful? Is it more than we would expect by chance just from sampling variation? We discuss these types of questions in this chapter.

Ratio Measures

One way to quantify the magnitude of difference between two measures of disease occurrence is by taking their ratio.

Risk Ratio

When we take the ratio of two risks, the numerator is a quantity separate from the denominator. In the numerator, we use the conditional risk of disease among the exposed; and in the denominator, we use the conditional risk of disease among the unexposed.

To illustrate the risk ratio, we return to an example from Chapter 5 of condom use and the risk of trichomoniasis. Recall that we have a sample of 20 individuals followed for 1 year with no loss to follow-up, 10 of whom are condom users.

We estimated the conditional risks of trichomoniasis among those exposed (non-condom users) and those not exposed (condom users) at 80% and 50%, respectively.

To estimate the risk ratio, we simply divide these conditional risks:

$$\text{Risk ratio} = \frac{80\%}{50\%} = 1.60$$

Therefore, individuals who do not use condoms in the sample had 1.6 times the risk of trichomoniasis over 1 year compared with individuals who used condoms.

Note that in the interpretation of the risk ratio, we should always include the time period of measurement (as we should when we estimate a risk, as discussed in Chapter 5). The ratio of risks for condom users compared with non-condom users is likely very different over 1 year than over 40 years. As such, the interpretation of the risk ratio is contingent on knowing the time period over which the risk was estimated.

Generalizing from this example, we formalize some notations for the 2 × 2 table in Figure 6.2.

As we move forward with formulas for measures of association and their associated confidence intervals, we are consistent using this notation, with the letter a denoting the number of individuals both exposed and having the health indicator; the letter b denoting the number of exposed without the health indicator; the letter c denoting the number of unexposed with the health indicator; and the letter d denoting the number of unexposed without the health indicator.

Thus, the general formula for the risk ratio is

$$\frac{\dfrac{a}{a+b}}{\dfrac{c}{c+d}},$$

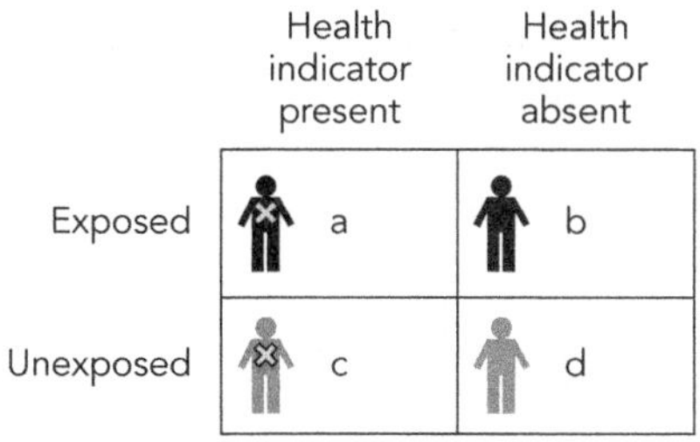

FIGURE 6.2 2 × 2 table notation.

Risk ratios can range from 0 to infinity. If there no increase or decrease in risk among exposed persons compared with unexposed, the risk ratio will be 1.0. If the risk of disease in the exposed is less than the risk of disease in the unexposed, the risk ratio will be less than 1.0; and conversely, a risk ratio greater than 1.0 indicates that the risk of disease is higher among exposed compared with unexposed.

The 95% Confidence Interval for a Risk Ratio

By chance, we may have selected a sample that does not represent the disease and exposure experience of the underlying population to which we wish to infer. Confidence intervals, as described in Chapter 5, can help us to understand the variability possible in our study estimates due to chance in the sampling process. Note that it is common in epidemiologic studies to see *p* values associated with measures of association. See Box 6.1 in the online material that accompanies Chapter 6 for our take on the *p* value and why we do not cover *p* values or hypothesis tests in this text.

As with our measures of disease occurrence, the key to estimating a confidence interval for a measure of association is estimating the standard error of the measure. Once we have the standard error, we can easily calculate the 90%, 95%, 99%, and so forth confidence interval for the risk ratio.

To estimate the standard error, we need to first transform the risk ratio to the natural log scale because the sampling distribution of the natural log of the risk ratio is approximately normal (see Box 5.2 in the online material that accompanies Chapter 6 for further explanation of the natural log).

Step 1: Take the natural log of the risk ratio

$$\text{Ln}\left(\text{Risk ratio}\right).$$

Second, we estimate the standard error. Note that this is the standard error for the natural log of the risk ratio.

Step 2: Estimate the standard error of the log of the risk ratio

$$\sqrt{\left(\frac{1}{a}\right)-\left(\frac{1}{a+b}\right)+\left(\frac{1}{c}\right)-\left(\frac{1}{c+d}\right)}.$$

Step 3: Estimate upper and lower bound for a confidence interval on the natural log scale

To accomplish this step, we first multiply the standard error for the natural log of the risk ratio and the appropriate z score. (For example, for a 95% confidence interval, the z score of interest is 1.96.) We then subtract this product from the sample natural log of the risk ratio to obtain a lower bound for the interval and add this product to the sample natural log of the risk ratio to obtain an upper bound for the interval.

Upper bound of 95% confidence interval of the log risk ratio is.

$$\mathrm{Ln}\left(\mathrm{Risk\ ratio}\right)+1.96\left(SE\left[\mathrm{ln}\left[\mathrm{Risk\ ratio}\right]\right]\right).$$

Lower bound of 95% confidence interval of the log risk ratio is

$$\mathrm{Ln}\left(\mathrm{Risk\ ratio}\right)-1.96\left(SE\left[\mathrm{ln}\left[\mathrm{Risk\ ratio}\right]\right]\right).$$

Step 4: Take the antilogarithm to obtain the upper and lower bounds of the confidence interval

Because we estimated the confidence interval on the natural log scale, the final step in determining the confidence interval on the original scale is to raise the natural number e to the upper and lower bounds (see Box 6.2 in the online material that accompanies this chapter for more description on why we use the natural log and its relation to e). Raising a value to the power of e is known as taking the antilogarithm of the value.

Lower bound of the 95% confidence interval of the risk ratio is

$$e^{\mathrm{Ln}\left(\mathrm{Risk\ ratio}\right)-1.96\left(SE\left[\mathrm{ln}\left[\mathrm{Risk\ ratio}\right]\right]\right)}.$$

Upper bound of the 95% confidence interval of the risk ratio is

$$e^{\mathrm{Ln}\left(\mathrm{Risk\ ratio}\right)+1.96\left(SE\left[\mathrm{ln}\left[\mathrm{Risk\ ratio}\right]\right]\right)}.$$

Step 5: Report and interpret the estimate and the confidence interval

The point estimate and confidence interval should be reported as follows: In these data, the exposed individuals had [risk ratio estimate] times the risk of the outcome compared with the unexposed, with a 95% confidence interval for the underlying population risk ratio ranging from [lower bound] to [upper bound]. The confidence interval can be interpreted as reflecting the statistical precision with which we can estimate the underlying population risk ratio.

We note that the underlying assumption for the validity of the confidence interval reflecting the true underlying risk ratio is that measurements are error free and groups are comparable. In epidemiology, this is unlikely to be the case. Therefore, although this is part of the statistical canon articulated in almost all introductory texts, we caution against an interpretation that the true population risk ratio lies within the bounds of the confidence interval with 95% confidence. We are only accounting for random variation in the sampling process with the 95% confidence interval; errors in measurement as well as any non-comparability between exposed and unexposed in the study sample will not be reflected in the confidence interval that is estimated. We provide an empiric example of a constructing a 95% confidence interval for a risk ratio in Box 6.3 of the online material that accompanies this chapter.

Assumptions for the CLT and Confidence Intervals

Remember that the validity of the confidence interval rests on the CLT, which holds only when sample sizes are large. For all of the confidence intervals and hypothesis tests discussed in this chapter, we must be able to show that the cell sizes or expected cell sizes of the 2×2 table (a, b, c, and d) are large enough for the CLT to hold and the confidence interval to be valid. There are many different rules of thumb that are used to judge whether the CLT holds. In general, the CLT will hold if each of the cell sizes or expected cell sizes in the 2×2 table contain at least 5 observations. Therefore, even in a sample that has a total size of, for example, 100,000 individuals, if only 3 of those individuals have the disease, then the CLT would not hold and one would want to be cautious about interpreting confidence intervals and other large-sample statistics. For example, it would be unwise to estimate a confidence interval for the trichomoniasis study discussed earlier in this chapter, as we only have 2 individuals who are exposed but did not develop trichomoniasis.

Rate Ratios

Risk ratios are accurate measures of association when there is little loss to follow-up. In most prospectively followed samples, however, there is substantial loss to follow-up. In those circumstances, the rate of disease is a more accurate representation of the incidence (see Chapter 5 for a discussion of rates). The rate ratio is a measure of association that compares two rates. In Figure 6.3, we add a column to the standard 2 × 2 table with the person years of observation among the exposed and the person years of observation among the unexposed. The rate ratio is estimated as follows:

$$\text{Rate of disease in the exposed} = \frac{a}{\text{person years exposed}}.$$

$$\text{Rate of disease in the unexposed} = \frac{c}{\text{person years unexposed}}.$$

The interpretation of the rate ratio is similar to the risk ratio in that ratios above 1.0 indicate that the rate is higher among exposed than among unexposed, ratios that are at 1.0 indicate no association, and rate ratios that are below 1.0 indicate that the rate is lower among exposed than among unexposed.

The 95% Confidence Interval for a Rate Ratio

The steps for estimating a 95% confidence interval for a rate ratio are similar to a risk ratio, with a different calculation for standard error:

Step 1: Take the natural log of the rate ratio

$$\text{Ln}\left(\text{Rate ratio}\right)$$

	Health indicator present	Health indicator absent	**Total**	Person years exposed
Exposed	a	b	a+b	Person years exposed
Unexposed	c	d	c+d	Person years unexposed
Total	a+c	b+d	Total population	Total person years

FIGURE 6.3 2 × 2 table with person years.

Step 2: Estimate the standard error of the log of the rate ratio

$$\sqrt{\left(\frac{1}{a}\right)+\left(\frac{1}{c}\right)}$$

Step 3: Estimate upper and lower bound confidence intervals on the log scale

$$Ln\left(\text{Rate ratio}\right)\pm 1.96 * SE\left(Ln\left[\text{Rate ratio}\right]\right)$$

Step 4: Take the antilogarithm to obtain the upper and lower bounds of the confidence interval

Lower bound of the 95% confidence interval of the rate ratio:

$$e^{Ln\left(\text{Rate ratio}\right)-1.96\left(SE\left[\ln\left[\text{Rate ratio}\right]\right]\right)}$$

Upper bound of the 95% confidence interval of the risk ratio:

$$e^{Ln\left(\text{Rate ratio}\right)+1.96\left(SE\left[\ln\left[\text{Rate ratio}\right]\right]\right)}$$

Step 5: Report and interpret the estimate and the confidence interval

The point estimate and confidence interval should be reported as follows: In these data, the exposed individuals had [rate ratio estimate] times the rate of the outcome compared with the exposed, with a 95% confidence interval for the population rate ratio ranging from [lower bound] to [upper bound].

We do not detail an example of confidence interval estimation for a rate ratio, as the process and interpretation are similar to the risk ratio we described earlier in this chapter.

Odds Ratios

The final commonly used measure of association in epidemiologic studies is the odds ratio. We use the odds ratio principally when we sample individuals with and without the health indicator of interest and retrospectively assess exposure status. We do this because the risk and rate ratios are not interpretable as measures of interest to us, but we can still obtain a reasonable estimate of the underlying risk ratio in the population base that gave rise to the cases with an odds ratio. To understand why, consider an example.

We are interested in whether smoking cigarettes during pregnancy is a potential cause of offspring attention deficit hyperactivity disorder (ADHD). We conduct a study of this association in Farrlandia. Some data suggest (although this is debated; Rowland et al., 2001) that the population prevalence of ADHD in many high-income countries is between 3% and 5%. We sample 500 10-year-old children in Farrlandia who are seeking care from their primary care physicians for ADHD. For each child with ADHD, we select 2 children of the same age from the same physician offices who present for routine well visits (i.e., do not have ADHD). Note that this is not a random sample but instead a purposive sample. As described in Chapter 4, this study design is often referred to as a case control study. We ask the mothers a series of questions, including whether they smoked cigarettes while they were pregnant. Our findings about the association between smoking during pregnancy and offspring ADHD among 1,500 mothers and children in Farrlandia are shown in Figure 6.4.

We expect that approximately 3%–5% of children in Farrlandia have ADHD. What is the prevalence of ADHD in our sample? It is 500 out of a total of 1,500 children sampled, or 33.3%. This is much higher than the estimated prevalence in the population! In fact, it is 33.3% by design. We, the investigators, decided to sample 500 children with the disorder and 1,000 children without the disorder, so the prevalence of ADHD in the sample is not a parameter that has any relation to a real population parameter. In other words, the prevalence of ADHD in the sample is not an estimate of the prevalence of ADHD in the population. Similarly, the conditional risk of ADHD (the risk of ADHD among those who smoked in pregnancy) is not a good estimate of the conditional risk in the population. Thus, risk ratios are inappropriate to estimating the association between pregnancy smoking and offspring ADHD in this study. Rate ratios are also not directly calculable in this study design, as we do not have information on the person time of follow-up. This example illustrates a more general concept—risk and rate ratios are not applicable when we cannot estimate longitudinal follow-up information within the sample.

	Health indicator present	Health indicator absent	Total N
Exposed	300	503	803
Unexposed	200	497	697
Total N	500	1000	1500

FIGURE 6.4 Association between smoking during pregnancy and offspring ADHD.

Rather, the measure of association most appropriate in this circumstance is an odds ratio. To understand why, we take a step back from the study just described. Suppose, instead of the study described, we conducted a cohort study. We recruit 5,000 women in Farrlandia during pregnancy who are smokers, and 5,000 women during pregnancy who are not smokers. We then assess their offspring at age 10 and determine which children developed ADHD and which did not. We assume that there was no loss to follow-up in this sample. Figure 6.5 contains the 2 × 2 table of the results.

First, we estimate the incidence proportion of ADHD in this sample. We have a total of 500 children with ADHD out of a total of 10,000 assessed across the exposed and unexposed group. Thus, the incidence proportion of ADHD is 500/10,000 = 0.05 or 5%, which is in line with previous research regarding the average incidence of ADHD in this age group. Now we estimate the risk ratio:

$$\frac{\dfrac{a}{a+b}}{\dfrac{c}{c+d}}$$

$$\text{Risk ratio} = \frac{\dfrac{300}{300+4700}}{\dfrac{200}{200+4800}} = 1.50$$

Offspring of women who smoked in pregnancy have 1.5 times the risk of developing ADHD over 10 years compared to offspring of women who did not smoke in pregnancy.

	Health indicator present	Health indicator absent	Total N
Exposed	300	4700	5000
Unexposed	200	4800	5000
Total N	500	9500	10000

FIGURE 6.5 Prospective study of the association between smoking during pregnancy and ADHD offspring.

Now, instead of the risk ratio, we calculate the odds ratio for the association. In Box 6.4 of the online material that accompanies this chapter, we provide an overview of the estimation of the odds. Similar to the risk and the rate ratio, an odds ratio is the ratio of two odds.

A general formula for estimating an odds ratio is

$$
\frac{\dfrac{\dfrac{a}{a+c}}{1-\left(\dfrac{a}{a+c}\right)}}{\dfrac{\dfrac{b}{b+d}}{1-\left(\dfrac{b}{b+d}\right)}}.
$$

or

$$
\frac{\dfrac{\dfrac{a}{a+b}}{1-\left(\dfrac{a}{a+b}\right)}}{\dfrac{\dfrac{c}{c+d}}{1-\left(\dfrac{c}{c+d}\right)}}
$$

The formula we use for the odds ratio depends on whether we are interested in the odds of exposure conditional on the presence or absence of the health indicator of interest or the odds of the health indicator conditional on the presence or absence of the exposure.

For our prospective study of maternal smoking and ADHD, we take the ratio of two odds: the odds of ADHD in the exposed (women who smoked in pregnancy) and the odds of ADHD in the unexposed (women who did not smoke in pregnancy).

Odds of ADHD among those exposed:

$$
\frac{\left(\dfrac{300}{5000}\right)}{1-\left(\dfrac{300}{5000}\right)} = 0.064.
$$

Odds of ADHD among those unexposed:

$$\frac{\left(\dfrac{200}{5000}\right)}{1-\left(\dfrac{200}{5000}\right)}=0.042.$$

Odds ratio:

$$\frac{0.064}{0.042}=1.52.$$

The interpretation of the odds ratio is that the odds of developing ADHD in the first 10 years of life among those exposed are 1.52 times the odds of disease in the unexposed.

Note that the odds ratio (1.52) is very close to the risk ratio (1.5). This is very important! Thus, we obtained a good estimate of the risk ratio for the association between exposure and the health indicator without using the risk ratio but instead using the odds ratio.

But why does this matter, if we can estimate the risk ratio directly in the cohort study? It matters because the relation between the risk ratio and the odds ratio has relevance for our ability to evaluate associations in the case control study where we cannot estimate the risk ratio directly.

Now we return to the original case control study. We cannot estimate risk directly. What we can estimate, however, is the proportion exposed among those who have the health indicator and among those who do not have the health indicator. Because we can estimate the prevalence of exposure among those with and without the health indicator, we can also estimate the odds of exposure among those with and without the health indicator.

Odds of exposure among those with ADHD:

$$\frac{\left(\dfrac{300}{500}\right)}{1-\left(\dfrac{300}{500}\right)}=1.5.$$

Odds of exposure among those without ADHD:

$$\frac{\left(\dfrac{503}{1000}\right)}{1-\left(\dfrac{503}{1000}\right)}=1.01.$$

Odds ratio in the case control study:

$$\frac{1.5}{1.01} = 1.49.$$

The strict interpretation of this measure is that the odds of exposure (mother smoking in pregnancy) among those with ADHD are 1.49 times higher among cases than among controls. We see that the odds ratio in the case control study is similar to the odds ratio that we got in the cohort study (1.49 vs. 1.52). Thus, we obtain a reasonably good estimate of the association between exposure and health indicator even though we were not able to directly estimate population parameters corresponding to the risk of the health indicator. This property makes the odds ratio a very useful measure in epidemiological studies that do not prospectively follow samples forward in time.

There are two additional important points worth considering regarding the odds ratio.

First, in our case control study, we estimated the odds of exposure given disease and the odds of exposure given no disease, then took the ratio. We call this the exposure odds ratio. It turns out, however, that the disease odds ratio (the ratio of the odds of disease given exposure and the odds of disease given no exposure) is mathematically equivalent to the exposure odds ratio (see Box 6.5 in the online material that accompanies Chapter 6). Second, in our example we were able to directly compare the results of a prospective study in which individuals were sampled based on exposure status to that of a case control study in which individuals were sampled based on disease status. In reality, we would hardly ever be able to do this type of comparison because we would not conduct both studies. We typically conduct a case control study when it is not efficient to conduct a long-term prospective study. We never know whether the odds ratio from the case control study is actually similar to the risk ratio we would have gotten from a prospective study. Two factors make these estimates diverge in some cases. The first is if the disease risk is high in the underlying population that gave rise to the cases. We cannot empirically know this based on our case control study because we set the number with and without disease. However, there might be other sources of data that we can use to estimate what we believe to be the general underlying risk. For example, for disorders such as obesity, with prevalence rising between 30%–40% in some areas of the United States (Ogden, Carroll, Kit, & Flegal, 2012), the odds ratio would not be a good approximation of the risk ratio.

Second, the odds ratio is not a good approximation of the risk ratio if the exposed and the unexposed in our case control study are not comparable on non-exposure factors related to disease. We delve into this topic in more detail in Chapters 8–10, but for now it is important to keep in mind that the selection of cases and controls into our study can potentially affect the magnitude of the odds ratio and thus the interpretation.

The 95% Confidence Interval for the Odds Ratio

Similar to other ratio measures, the standard error for an odds ratio is estimated on the log scale. Thus, the steps for estimating a 95% confidence interval are as follows:

Step 1: Take the natural log of the odds ratio

$$Ln\left(\text{Odds ratio}\right)$$

Step 2: Estimate the standard error of the log of the odds ratio

$$\sqrt{\left(\frac{1}{a}\right)+\left(\frac{1}{b}\right)+\left(\frac{1}{c}\right)+\left(\frac{1}{d}\right)}$$

Step 3: Estimate upper and lower bound confidence intervals on the log scale

$$Ln\left(\text{Odds ratio}\right)\pm 1.96 * SE\left(Ln\left[\text{Odds ratio}\right]\right)$$

Step 4: Take the antilogarithm to obtain the upper and lower bounds of the confidence interval

Lower bound of the 95% confidence interval of the odds ratio:

$$e^{Ln\left(\text{Odds ratio}\right)-1.96\left(SE\left[\ln\left[\text{Odds ratio}\right]\right]\right)}$$

Upper bound of the 95% confidence interval of the odds ratio:

$$e^{Ln\left(\text{Odds ratio}\right)+1.96\left(SE\left[\ln\left[\text{Odds ratio}\right]\right]\right)}$$

Step 5: Report and interpret the estimate and the confidence interval

The point estimate and confidence interval should be reported as follows: In these data, the exposed individuals had [odds ratio estimate] times the odds of the outcome compared with the unexposed, with a 95% confidence interval for the population odds ratio ranging from [lower bound] to [upper bound].

We do not detail an example of confidence interval estimation for an odds ratio, as the process and interpretation are similar to the risk ratio we described previously in this chapter.

Summary

We cannot estimate the risk of disease directly when we sample people based on whether they have the health indicator or not (the case control study). However, we can estimate the proportion who are exposed among those both with and without the health indicator. With this proportion, we can estimate the odds ratio for exposure. The odds ratio for exposure is equivalent to the odds ratio for disease. Under certain conditions, the odds ratio will approximate the risk ratio that we would have gotten if we had done a prospective study in which risk could be directly estimated (assuming no non-comparability in our case control study, to be discussed in Chapter 9). Thus, the odds ratio from the case control study is a very useful measure.

Difference Measures

Thus far we have discussed ratio measures, including the risk ratio, rate ratio, and odds ratio. Ratio measures divide one measure by another. Whereas ratio measures are standard in epidemiology, difference measures are also frequently used and important measures for estimating public health risk. There is no reason to think that one set of measures is any better than the other and both have their own uses. We use both ratio and difference measures in examples going forward. Note that difference between two odds is not a measure with any valuable interpretation in epidemiologic studies; thus, we focus on the risk difference and the rate difference.

Risk Difference

The risk difference is quite literally the difference between two risks. It is estimated as

$$\left(\frac{a}{a+b}\right) - \left(\frac{c}{c+d}\right)$$

We understand the interpretation of a risk difference through an example. We conduct a study in Farrlandia of whether nutrition classes in middle school are associated with the development of obesity in adolescence. One middle school composed of 400 students receives the health education. Another middle school in a neighboring district does not have nutrition class and is composed of 300 students. Each year the school records the students' height and weight, which we are able to obtain. Thus, this is a purposive sample in that the students are not drawn from a random sample of all possible middle schools. While studying the association between middle school nutrition class and incidence of obesity among 700 students in Farrlandia across 5 years, we obtain the data described in Figure 6.6.

The risk of obesity among those who had nutrition class is 0.18 or 18%. The risk of obesity among those who did not have nutrition class is 0.33 or 33%. Therefore, the risk difference is

$$\text{Risk difference} : 0.18 - 0.33 = -0.15$$

How do we interpret this measure? We can conceptualize this as indicating that there are approximately 15 fewer cases (-0.15×100) of obesity during adolescence for every 100 students who had the nutrition class compared with those who did not have the nutrition class.

The 95% Confidence Interval for the Risk Difference

In contrast to the confidence interval for ratio measures, we do not need to estimate the standard error for the natural log of the measure. Instead, we can estimate the standard error for the risk difference directly.

	Health indicator present	Health indicator absent	Total N
Exposed	70	330	400
Unexposed	100	200	300
Total N	170	530	700

FIGURE 6.6 Association between middle school nutrition class and incidence of obesity.

Step 1: Estimate the standard error for the risk difference

$$\sqrt{\frac{a*b}{(a+b)^3} + \frac{c*d}{(c+d)^3}}.$$

Step 2: Estimate upper and lower bound confidence intervals

$$\text{Risk difference} \pm 1.96 * SE\left(\text{Risk difference}\right).$$

Step 3: Report and interpret the estimate and the confidence interval

If the risk difference is positive, we would interpret as follows: In these data, exposure was associated with an excess of [risk difference estimate * 100] cases per 100 exposed compared with unexposed, with a 95% confidence interval for the excess cases ranging in the population from [lower bound] to [upper bound]. Note that a risk difference of 0 indicates that there is no difference in risk between exposed and unexposed.

If the risk difference is negative, we would interpret as follows: In these data, exposure was associated with an [risk difference estimate * 100] fewer cases per 100 exposed compared with the unexposed, with a 95% confidence interval for the decrease in cases in the population ranging from [lower bound] to [upper bound].

Example of Estimating a 95% Confidence Interval for a Risk Difference

As an example, we use the data described in the section titled "Risk Difference." The estimated risk difference in the sample was −0.155.

Standard error of the risk difference:

$$\sqrt{\frac{70*330}{(70+330)^3} + \frac{100*200}{(100+200)^3}} = 0.03.$$

The upper bound of the confidence interval is thus

$$-0.15 + \left(1.96 * 0.03\right) = -0.09.$$

The lower bound of the confidence interval is thus

$$-0.155 - \left(1.96 * 0.03\right) = -0.21.$$

There are approximately 15 fewer cases of obesity during adolescence among those who had the nutrition class compared with those who did not have the nutrition class, with a 95% confidence interval for the observed decrease in cases from 9 to 21 fewer cases.

Rate Difference

The rate difference is estimated similarly to the risk difference, only now we use rates instead of risks:

$$\left(\frac{a}{\text{person years exposed}} \right) - \left(\frac{c}{\text{person years unexposed}} \right).$$

The interpretation of the rate difference is also similar to that of the risk difference. It is the excess rate associated with the exposure. For example, if the rate of disease is 8 per 100,000 person years in the unexposed and 4 per 100,000 person years in the exposed, then 4 additional cases per 100,000 exposed is associated with the exposure of interest.

The 95% Confidence Interval for a Rate Difference

Similar to the risk difference, we do not need to estimate the standard error on the natural log scale and can estimate the standard error directly for the rate difference.

Step 1: Estimate the standard error for the rate difference

$$\sqrt{\left(\frac{a}{PY_1^{\,2}} \right) + \left(\frac{c}{PY_2^{\,2}} \right)}$$

Where PY_1 is the total person time contributed among exposed, and PY_2 is the total person time contributed among the unexposed.

Step 2: Estimate upper and lower bound confidence intervals

$$\text{Rate difference} \pm 1.96 * SE\left(\text{Rate difference}\right)$$

Step 3: Report and interpret the estimate and the confidence interval

If the rate difference is positive, we would interpret as follows: In these data, exposure was associated with an increase of [rate difference estimate] per 100 person years of exposure compared with the unexposed, with a 95% confidence interval for the population excess rate ranging from [lower bound] to [upper bound].

If the rate difference is negative, we would interpret as follows: In these data, exposure was associated with an decrease of [rate difference estimate] per 100 person years of exposure compared with the unexposed, with a 95% confidence interval for the population decrease in the rate ranging from [lower bound] to [upper bound]. As with the risk difference, a rate difference of 0 indicates no difference in the rate between exposed and unexposed.

We do not detail an example of confidence interval estimation for a rate difference, as the process and interpretation are similar to the risk difference we described earlier in this chapter.

Risk/Rate Differences Versus Risk/Rate Ratios

When is a ratio measure more appropriate than a difference measure? Why would we use one over the other? These measures provide different information and are appropriate in different contexts. Difference measures provide a gauge of the potential direct public health benefit of intervention, whereas ratio measures provide an intuitive summary of the magnitude of differences in two exposures.

Consider the following two studies. Study 1 is estimating the association between exposure A and disease Y among 100 study participants. Study 2 is estimating the association between exposure B and disease Z among a different 100 study participants. Both studies are across 1 year.

STUDY 1:
Risk of disease Y among exposed to A: 4%
Risk of disease Y among unexposed to A: 2%

$$\text{Risk ratio}: \frac{.04}{.02} = 2.0.$$

The risk of disease across 1 year among exposed is 2.0 times that of the unexposed.

$$\text{Risk difference}: 0.04-0.02 = 0.02.$$

There are an additional 2 cases of disease across 1 year per 100 persons exposed compared with unexposed.

STUDY 2:

Risk of disease Z among exposed to B: 60%

Risk of disease Z among unexposed to B: 30%

$$\text{Risk ratio}: \frac{.06}{.03} = 2.0$$

The risk of disease across 1 year among exposed is 2.0 times that of the unexposed.

$$\text{Risk difference}: 0.6 - 0.3 = 0.30$$

There are an additional 30 cases of disease across 1 year per 100 persons exposed compared with unexposed.

In both studies, the risk of the disease among the exposed is 2.0 times that of the unexposed. But the risk differences vary widely. For every 100 people, there are 30 cases of disease associated with Exposure B and just 2 excess cases of disease associated with Exposure A in 1 year. In terms of public health planning, this is vital information to have, as the burden of disease will be much greater for Exposure B on disease Z. In summary, both ratio and difference measures should be estimated and reported as appropriate in epidemiologic studies.

Population Attributable Risk Proportion

One final measure of association that is often reported in epidemiologic studies is known as the population attributable risk proportion (PARP). The PARP is also sometimes termed the population attributable fraction. The PARP is a measure of the amount of the total disease burden that is associated with the exposure of interest. Consider our first example in this chapter, the proportion of people who develop heart disease among smokers and nonsmokers. The risk of heart disease in the smokers was 14%, and the risk of the disease in the nonsmokers was 5%. The PARP would be calculated as follows:

$$PARP = \frac{\left(\dfrac{a}{a+b}\right) - \left(\dfrac{c}{c+d}\right)}{\dfrac{a}{a+b}}$$

$$\frac{14 - 5}{14} = 0.64$$

The interpretation would be that 64% of heart disease cases in the population of Farrlandia are potentially attributable to smoking. Alternatively, we could also interpret this measure as suggesting that if we were to convince all of the smokers to quit, we would reduce the risk of heart disease by 64%. This measure is sometimes considered particularly useful in public health practice where it may help suggest useful directions for policy.

There are several key limitations of the PARP as a measure of association. First, if we were to sum the PARP for most common exposures for any outcome, the result would be much greater than 100% because often these exposures interact with each other (see Chapter 11). Second, the PARP assumes a causal relation (see Chapter 7) between the exposure and outcome to be interpretable. Thus, 64% of heart disease is attributable to smoking only to the extent that smoking actually causes heart disease.

Summary

In this chapter, we finish describing Step 3 of the seven-step summary of fundamentals for conducting epidemiologic studies, which is estimating a quantitative measure of the association between exposure and a health indicator of interest. As we discussed in Chapter 3, exposures can be broadly defined; in this chapter, our exposures ranged from interventions to prenatal insults to health behaviors. Regardless of the hypothesized factor related to the outcome, developing and estimating quantitative measures that describe the strength of an exposure–health indicator relation is a fundamental aspect of epidemiologic studies. In this chapter, we described how to estimate risk ratios, rate ratios, odds ratios, risk differences, and rate differences and their confidence intervals. We also described when each measure is appropriate in various sampling strategies from an underlying population base. Armed with knowledge about the association between an exposure and a health indicator, the next step is to rigorously assess whether the observed relation reflects a causal relation, which we detail beginning in Chapter 7.

References

Ogden, C. L., Carroll, M. D., Kit, B. K., & Flegal, K. M. (2012). Prevalence of obesity in the United States, 2009–2010. *NCHS Data Brief, 82*, 1–8.

Rowland, A. S., Umbach, D. M., Catoe, K. E., Stallone, L., Long, S., . . . Sandler, D. P. (2001). Studying the epidemiology of attention-deficit hyperactivity disorder: screening method and pilot results. *Canadian Journal of Psychiatry, 46*, 931–940.

7

What Is a Cause?

IDENTIFYING FACTORS THAT cause disease is the central driving force behind the discipline of epidemiology. We design studies, carefully construct measures, take samples, and follow individuals over time to identify true causes of disease and design interventions to prevent these causes from exerting a negative influence on health. Following our seven steps toward an epidemiology of consequence, we now approach Step 5 in which we rigorously assess whether the associations observed in our data reflect casual associations of exposures on health indicators. To properly design studies that will identify causes of disease, we first must ask—what is a cause?

In this chapter, we articulate a framework for how to conceptualize causes of disease across the life course and within interconnected networks of individuals. Understanding the concept of a cause is not a definitional but rather a philosophical endeavor. Causal effects are inferred from our data but are never directly observed. We rely on a combination of theory, design, and triangulation of research evidence across multiple studies to infer whether the weight of the evidence favors the exposure as a cause of the health indicator. With that in mind, in this chapter we articulate a conceptual architecture for causal thinking that may usefully guide how we interpret observed associations across studies with diverse designs and samples.

A Motivating Example of Multifactorial Causation

Uncle Joe smoked a pack of cigarettes every day, consumed copious amounts of alcohol, ate greasy bacon and eggs every morning and steak every evening, and eschewed any type of food that was green and from the earth. Yet despite exemplifying almost every unhealthy behavior one can imagine, Uncle Joe lived to be 102, and by all accounts did not suffer any major health disability during his long tenure on earth. How can cigarette smoking, excessive alcohol consumption, and unhealthy diet be causes of disease when some people smoke their entire lives, drink excessively, and eat terribly yet never seem to develop any illness related to their health behaviors?

Although the Uncle Joe example may perhaps be extreme, rationalization through anecdote is rampant in our daily lives and in the media. For example, we have all likely heard someone say, "My mother smoked in pregnancy—no one knew the health dangers back then—and I am just fine. All of these warnings about smoking during pregnancy are overdone." If one person remains healthy after his or her mother smoked during pregnancy, does this mean that in utero exposure to cigarettes cannot be a cause of adverse health outcomes later in life? More broadly, if some people live unscathed after being exposed to a factor believed to be involved in the disease causation process, is that factor not a cause of disease? In this chapter, we explain how epidemiologists understand disease causation to be a multifactorial process and how this offers us a framework that we can use to understand why the observation that smoking is a cause of disease is not incompatible with Uncle Joe living to 102.

What Is a Cause?

Scholars from many disciplines have provided us with excellent definitions of cause. In short, and for our purposes, we draw on definitions elaborated by Rothman (Rothman 2008; also, Rothman & Greenland, 2005) as well as Schwartz and Susser (2006) and consider a cause to be a factor that contributes, at least in part, to the development of illness, at least in some individuals. We provide some historical context for the evolution of causal inference in epidemiology in Box 7.1 of the online material that accompanies Chapter 7.

To understand how epidemiologists conceptualize causes of disease, consider the following scenario. A man developed depression last year. When reviewing his history, we are told the following: He was born in Boise, Idaho, in 1965. His parents were manual laborers, and he is the youngest of five children. The family lived in a modest three-bedroom home. In adolescence, the man acted out, had difficulty concentrating, and was in trouble at school and with the law on a regular basis. He began working at a manufacturing plant after graduating from high school. He did not attend college. He was married at age 25 and had one child at age 28. Four years ago, his wife filed for divorce, citing his heavy drinking as a principal reason for the split. Two years ago the plant he had been working at since age 18 shut down, and he has been unable to find another job since then. His heavy drinking has continued throughout this time period.

What Are the Causes of the Man's Depression?

It seems logical that the loss of his job, which is the event most proximal (i.e., closest in time) to the onset of the depressive symptoms, is likely involved. The divorce was likely also a stressful event that may have contributed to the depression; we might hypothesize that there is no longer the same social support structure in place to mitigate the stress of the job loss. The man is also a heavy drinker, which may contribute to symptoms of depression. What about childhood? It seems that the man grew up with limited resources, which may have affected parental supervision (leading to trouble with the law) or difficulty concentrating, all of which may be implicated in the propensity to develop depression. In sum, all of these factors could be involved in the onset of the depression. How do we decide which of these factors are causes of depression?

We can ask the question of each potential cause: Would the depression have occurred if we kept everything about the man's life the same but changed one detail? Here are three examples of these types of questions.

Example 1: If everything about the man stayed the same, but the plant had not closed, would the depression have occurred? If we believe the answer to be no, then the plant closing is a cause.

Example 2: If everything about the man had stayed the same, but the divorce had not occurred, would the depression have occurred? Regardless of the mechanistic link we think exists between divorce and depression (i.e., divorce can create a stressful home environment or remove social support that may have helped the man cope with the plant closing), if the depression would not have occurred in the absence of the divorce, all else being equal, the divorce is a cause of depression.

Example 3: If everything about the man had stayed the same, but more resources were available in his childhood, would the depression have occurred? This one is trickier, because the cascade of his life circumstances may have been changed substantially if more resources were available in childhood. Perhaps he would have been better able to focus in school, would have been in less trouble as an adolescent, may have attended college, and so forth. However, we would still posit childhood resources as a cause of depression if the depression would not have occurred exactly how and when it did in the presence of more material resources during his childhood.

These questions—"if everything had stayed the same except one thing changed . . . "—are an example of counterfactual thinking. Simply put, the counterfactual is the condition that is counter to the fact. If an individual has been exposed to a certain factor, that factor is a cause of disease for that individual if the same individual would not have developed the disease had the exposure not occurred or occurred differently (e.g., lower dose or later onset). We say a factor is a cause if the outcome would not have occurred in the absence of that factor, holding everything else constant, including space and time.

Disease Causation Illustrated Through a Game of Marbles

We now understand that the definition of a cause can be conceptualized through a counterfactual argument. An exposure causes a health indicator if, holding all else constant, the outcome would have been different if, contrary to the fact, an individual who was exposed had not been exposed. However, the counterfactual condition can never be observed because we cannot go back in time and manipulate exposures. That said, we can engage in a thought experiment about what would have happened if we were able to observe an individual or groups of individuals under the condition of being exposed and then of being not exposed.

It is important to note that we are still in the realm of a theoretical thought experiment. In the following section, we assume that we know all of the exposures that cause a particular health indicator and that we know whether every individual in the population is exposed or unexposed to these factors. In reality, we never know the full array of factors that cause health indicators, nor do we know every individual's exposure status to each factor; however, engaging in an exercise about what we would see if we could know all of the mechanics of disease causes is instructive. Underlying what we can observe is a causal architecture that is unobservable. By theoretically understanding the unobservable causal architecture that forms human disease, we can better design studies and interpret our findings.

Causes of a Disease in an Individual

We formalize the counterfactual questions posed previously in a more systematic theoretical framework, beginning with an individual and a disease. For each individual there is a set of exposures that caused a particular disease. Without any one of these exposures, the disease would not have occurred. Thus, each exposure fulfills the counterfactual question: "Would the disease have occurred when and how it did without this exposure?"

There is a further point that is critical, however. In most circumstances, not just one but several exposures must all be present for an individual to get the health outcome. A single cause does not produce the disease, but the combination of many causes produces the disease. This is what we mean when we talk about a multifactorial disease. When each exposure is necessary for the person to develop the health indicator, but no one exposure in and of itself is the sole cause, we say that the exposures are insufficient. They are each necessary but each insufficient to produce the outcome on their own.

Together, the set of exposures that, alone, are necessary but insufficient become a sufficient set of exposures that cause the health indicator in at least one person. Sufficient sets of exposures are those that produce the health indicator of interest.

We consider an example. Type II diabetes is a multifactorial disease that is increasingly prevalent worldwide. There are many different combinations of types of causes that can bring about diabetes in a person. Each exposure that is a potential cause of diabetes we call "component causes." Person 1 may be obese, have a lack of preventive care, have a family history of diabetes, and have 20 pack-years of smoking. Each of these is a component cause. In this person, all of these component causes are necessary for Type II diabetes to occur. If the individual were obese, had a family history of diabetes, and 20 pack-years of smoking but had regular preventive care, the diabetes would not have occurred for this individual. Similarly, if the individual were obese, lacked preventive care, and had 20 pack-years of smoking but did not have a family history of diabetes, then the diabetes would not have occurred. All four component causes therefore were necessary for disease to occur in that individual, but no component cause alone produced the disease; therefore, all were insufficient.

Person 2 may have another combination of component causes. These may be (a) lack of nutrition education, (b) family history of diabetes, (c) high blood pressure, and (d) advanced age. None of these component causes singularly produced disease (they were all insufficient alone), but all component causes worked together and disease occurred as a result (they were all sufficient together).

Person 3 may have another combination of component causes including (a) obesity, (b) family history of diabetes, and (c) high blood pressure. Although these factors were part of the sufficient cause of disease for Persons 1 or 2, they do not result in disease for Person 3. There are therefore other component causes that need to be collected, and as of yet have not been collected, before diabetes occurs for Person 3. Because the same component causes that were involved in disease for Persons 1 and 2 do not result in disease for Person 3, we know that the disease is multifactorial and that no one exposure or set of exposures are sufficient to produce the disease in all individuals.

To help conceptualize this, we present the idea of a game of marbles, drawing on the framework explicated by Rothman (see Box 7.1 in the online material that accompanies this chapter; see also Rothman, 1976; Rothman & Greenland, 2005). We imagine a disease, such as Type II diabetes, that has many different component causes. Each cause is individually a component that, together with other causes, produces the disease in an individual. Schematically we represent individuals with disease with an X and those without disease without the X. Each component cause is represented by a marble with a unique design (Figure 7.1). For example, there are different marbles for smoking (a component cause of Type II diabetes) and for obesity (another component cause of Type II diabetes).

Each individual has a jar. This jar represents the disease. Once the marbles fill the jar with a specific combination and frequency, the disease will occur. The marbles that fill the jar may be different for each individual, but every individual has a jar that will result in the disease if filled in a specific way. Therefore, the marbles each represent necessary causes, and the marble jars represent sufficient causes.

Following the previous example, Person 1 has four marbles in that individual's jar and is also diseased. All four of these marbles together caused disease (the X) in this individual, meaning that each component cause was a necessary cause for this individual; that is, the disease would not have occurred if

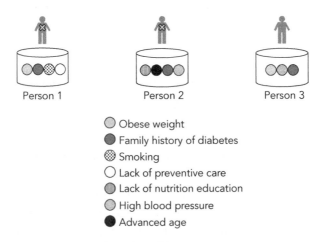

FIGURE 7.1 Disease causation through marbles in a jar.

the individual only had three marbles. No marble caused the disease alone, indicating that no component cause was a sufficient cause; the disease only occurred when all four marbles were present. Therefore, each marble was necessary and insufficient; the marble jar with four marbles represented a sufficient cause of the disease.

In Person 2, a different combination of four marbles together jointly produced the disease in the individual's marble jar; thus there were four component causes that produced disease in this individual. Similar to Person 1, if one marble were removed, the disease would not have occurred. Therefore, similar to Person 1, each marble was necessary but insufficient, and the four marbles together in the jar formed a sufficient cause. The sufficient cause for Person 2 was different from the sufficient cause for Person 1.

In Person 3, we see that although this person did have certain marbles, they did not have enough, or the right combination, to produce the disease. Perhaps 1, 2, or 10 additional marbles are needed for the disease process to initiate in this person. Therefore, this person did not have enough marbles to create a sufficient cause of disease.

Summary

In our marble analogy, we see that collections of marbles, or component causes, work jointly together to promote disease in individuals. A collection of marbles that work together to produce disease is a sufficient cause. Individuals may develop the same disease based on different combinations of marbles that form the sufficient cause (as in Person 1 and 2). Further, whereas some individuals may have some of the same marbles, some will have the disease and some will not depending on the other marbles in their marble jars (as in Person 1 and Person 3). These causes are rooted in a counterfactual definition: Each marble is a cause of disease if the individual would not have developed the disease without that marble. In Table 7.1, we provide some examples from the literature further explicating the relation between necessary and sufficient causes.

Disease at the Level of the Population

Although we have used individual causal frameworks to introduce the notions of component, necessary, and sufficient causes, epidemiology is a population science. Therefore, we never observe causal architecture at the individual level but rather at the population level. We have demonstrated thus far that

Table 7.1 Necessary and Sufficient Causes: Empiric Examples

Scenario	Example	Explanation
Necessary and sufficient causes	Trisomy 21 and Down Syndrome	All individuals with three copies of the 21st chromosome will show evidence of Down Syndrome (therefore, three copies of chromosome 21 is a sufficient cause in all cases). All individuals with Down syndrome have three copies of the 21st chromosome (therefore, three copies of chromosome 21 is a necessary cause in all cases).
Necessary but insufficient causes	Alcohol consumption and alcoholism	Not all individuals who consume alcohol will develop alcoholism (therefore, alcohol consumption is not a sufficient cause), but all individuals with alcoholism will have consumed alcohol (therefore, alcohol consumption is a necessary cause).
Unnecessary but sufficient cause	Hysterectomy and pregnancy prevention	All women who have a hysterectomy are unable to become pregnant (therefore, hysterectomy is sufficient to prevent pregnancy), but there are many other methods available to prevent pregnancy (therefore, hysterectomy is not necessary to prevent pregnancy).
Unnecessary and insufficient cause	Smoking and lung cancer	Individuals who smoke are at higher risk for lung cancer. Not all individuals who smoke will develop lung cancer (therefore, smoking is not sufficient to cause lung cancer), and some people with lung cancer are lifelong nonsmokers (therefore, smoking is not necessary to cause lung cancer).

individuals typically acquire disease from a series of component causes working together within the individual's marble jar. Now we extend this analogy to describe how disease processes at the individual level translate to describing population patterns of disease.

Although causes may be necessary and/or sufficient for any individual to acquire the health indicator of interest, in public health we are concerned with how many individuals are exposed to a certain cause of interest and how many of those individuals have potential component causes that would complete a marble jar.

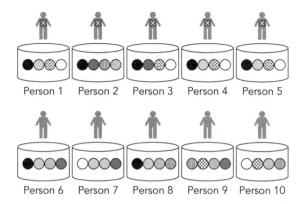

FIGURE 7.2 Causes of disease at the population level.

Consider the example in Figure 7.2. Here we have 10 individuals. Each individual has a jar filled with different combinations of marbles; 5 of the 10 individuals have the disease.

All individuals with the disease (marked with an X) have a black marble. Therefore, the black marble was necessary for the disease to occur in all individuals who developed the health indicator. If we remove the black marble from the population, we would eliminate disease. Notice, however, that two individuals without the disease have a black marble. Whereas the black marble is necessary for the disease to occur in all individuals, it is not sufficient to produce the disease in any individual. Consider the alcohol consumption and alcoholism: All individuals with alcoholism have consumed alcohol; therefore, it is necessary. If we were to remove all alcohol from the world, there would be no alcoholism. But not all individuals who consume alcohol will develop alcoholism; therefore, it is not sufficient.

Three of the five individuals with the disease have the same marble combination in their jar; that is, the same sufficient cause (i.e., a set of necessary component causes) produced the disease in three individuals. No other individuals in the population have this particular set of marbles; however, two individuals became diseased based on a different sufficient cause. Therefore, multiple sufficient causes exist within this population; there is not a single set of component causes that inevitably produce the disease. In practice, it is difficult to determine what sets of component causes will render a sufficient cause or how many individuals in the population acquired the disease from which exact sets of sufficient causes; however, the definition remains useful in conceptualizing how causes work together.

In summary, at the individual level we have marbles and marble jars. Marbles are causes that meet the counterfactual definition. They are necessary, but often insufficient, to produce health indicators in any one individual. Sets of marbles form marble jars and those that jointly work together to produce health indicators are sufficient causes. At the population level, we can conceptualize the frequency of these marbles across individuals. There may be causes that are present in every case of disease, in which case they are necessary for all individuals who develop the health indicator. Within a population, there may be many sufficient causes, and individuals who have the same health indicator may have developed the health indicator through a different set of sufficient causes.

It is important to remember that this exercise is theoretical. We rarely know what marble jars will be sufficient to cause disease and what specific sets of marbles are in each jar. However, underneath what we can observe is this causal architecture in which there are marble jars, or sets of causes, that are sufficient to produce disease.

Disease Causation Through Time and Space: Extending the Marble Analogy

Thus far we have used the analogy of marbles and marble jars to describe the process of disease causation. However, the model that we have described thus far, rooted heavily in the sufficient-component cause framework (Rothman, 1976; Rothman & Greenland, 2005), leaves unexplored some essential pieces of the disease causation process.

Collecting Marbles Across the Life Course

The onset of a disease happens at a specific moment in time, but the process of disease causation can begin much earlier than the time of disease onset. Health outcomes such as low birth weight originate in utero, with causes such as maternal smoking during pregnancy playing a critical role (Kramer, 1987). Accumulating evidence indicates that exposures such as maternal smoking, environmental toxins, diet and obesity, and other factors during gestation may impact lifelong health (we provide a seminal example of a disease process that begins in utero with the case of diethylstilbestrol and vaginal cancer in Box 7.2 of the online material that accompanies this chapter). The overarching principle of life course research is that health outcomes in adulthood may have tractable origins early in life and may be influenced by exposures occurring throughout the life course to produce disease in adulthood. Consider our earlier example of the man with depression. His early childhood influences may have had an impact on the development of depression in adulthood. He was essentially collecting marbles throughout his life that eventually led to depression in adulthood.

We illustrate this concept using our marble analogy in Figure 7.3. We have one individual progressing through the life course from birth to adolescence to young adulthood to older adulthood. Some marbles are present at birth, some are acquired at a single point, and some slowly accumulate over time. For example, this person had one marble prior to birth (the black marble at the top of Figure 7.3). This marble may represent exposure to tobacco smoke or other toxins in utero. He also acquired a series of grey marbles in childhood. These may represent ongoing exposures to chronic poverty, chaotic home environment, or low levels of parental support. In adolescence, he began being exposed to the white marble, which

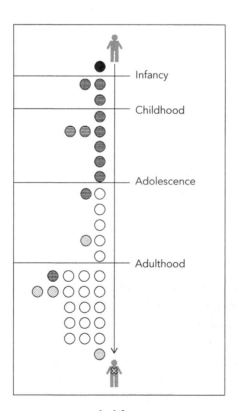

FIGURE 7.3 Collecting exposures over the life course.

accumulated yearly, with increasing amounts of exposure during adulthood. This might represent cigarette smoking, which begins for this individual in adolescence in a low dose and then increases in adulthood and remains a consistent exposure throughout his life. Additional marbles began accumulating during adulthood until disease onset at the bottom of Figure 7.3. Thus, each individual is slowly accumulating marbles as they move through the life course until disease onset.

The concepts we explicated in the previous section remain. Each marble in the jar produced disease when and how it did for this individual. Now, however, we make the case that marbles are accumulating within each individual all along the life course. Some component causes require a long duration of exposure to exert an impact; for example, smoking a single cigarette is unlikely to cause lung cancer, but prolonged heavy smoking for several decades is a component cause in many lung cancers. Some causes exert an impact due to when they occur; malnutrition during specific periods of gestation, for example, is associated with increased risk of mental health outcomes in adulthood (Lumey, Stein & Susser, 2011). Some component causes may produce other component causes; for example, poverty in childhood may lead to lower education in adulthood and lack of job opportunities.

Marbles May Be Dependent

Marbles can be shared between individuals and one person's marble collection may influence another person's marble collection. This is distinct from the concept of some people having the same marble in their jar (e.g., two individuals who are both obese); marbles can also be shared because one person's marble influences another person's disease status. The most dramatic way in which we see this concept is in person-to-person infectious disease transmission. When infectious diseases are transmitted between people (e.g., through salivary or skin-to-skin spread, genital contact, or from mother to child), one person's disease status becomes an exposure for those who are in direct contact with that person. Thus, the marbles are collected not only through the life course; they can also be shared among people as the disease is transmitted within and across communities. This concept of shared space in which exposures and outcomes do not occur independently but rather are dependent on shared exposures and outcomes in the community is a concept now being extended to noninfectious diseases as well. For example, some theories of depression suggest that living in a dense urban environment contributes to depressive symptoms

(Walters et al., 2004). The density of the population is not a character-istic of individuals; rather, it is a characteristic of the local environment that is based on the number of individuals and the size of the neighbor-hood. Thus, the population density of a specific area is shared among the individuals in that area. Similarly, community violence (Krug, Mercy, Dahlberg, & Zwi, 2002), social norms around substance use and cigarette smoking (Galea, Nandi, & Vlahov, 2004), and macro exposures such as policies and laws restricting access to quality health care (Zuber, 2012) are marbles that are shared across space and time. Evidence is even accumulat-ing that outcomes not traditionally conceived of as communicable from person to person may have transmissibility. For example, adolescents are more likely to begin smoking if an influential peer begins smoking (Urberg, Shyu, & Liang, 1990), and community samples of adults suggest that hav-ing obese friends increases the probability that an individual will develop obesity (Christakis & Fowler, 2007).

Thus, although transmission of disease across individuals because of an infectious agent or because of an exposure that is shared in the environment are distinct routes of disease etiology, the end result is the same in that indi-viduals are sharing marbles.

We illustrate this concept using the marble analogy in Figure 7.4. We have four people, two of whom have the disease. In contrast to ear-lier figures in this chapter, now all four people have circles around them, intersecting with other people. Some marbles are unique to the individ-ual. These unique marbles may be factors such as genetic predisposition, personal dietary intake of fiber, exercise behavior, and stressful life events such as divorce and job loss. Some are shared with other individuals. These shared marbles could correspond to causes from people who live in the same geographic area, are in the same family, are sexual partners or share sexual partners, or are connected in another way that allows for exposures to be shared between people.

The concepts of necessity and sufficiency that were introduced in the begin-ning of this chapter remain once we introduce the idea of shared marble space rather than specific marble jars. Within each individual's marble space, each cause was required for that individual to manifest the disease when and how they did. Some individuals (Persons 1 and 3) have collections of causes shared in their space, and some of these collections produce disease for all individuals who share this combination. Marbles can cross spaces and be shared among individuals such that a single cause maybe part of the constellation of marbles for many individuals.

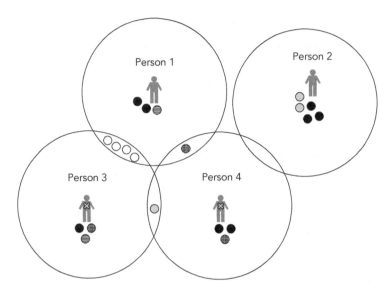

Each marble represents an exposure. Some marbles are shared between individuals; for example, Person 1 and Person 3 share four clear marbles, and Person 3 shares one grey marble with Person 4. Individuals also have marbles that are unique and unshared; for example, Person 1 has two black marbles that are unshared, as does Person 4. Examples of shared marbles could be neighborhoods, social norms, or sex partners. Examples of unique marbles could be genetic alleles, dietary patterns, and experiences of personal trauma.

FIGURE 7.4 Sharing marble exposure.

Summary

Exposure to unsafe or unhealthy environments as well as transmission of behavior and disease are extraordinarily important concepts for us to understand to effectively intervene and prevent adverse health conditions at the population level. We can understand this causal theory using the marble analogy in which individuals share marbles and/or transmit marbles from one space to another. One person's complete set of marbles may differ from another person's, as disease can manifest through multiple mechanisms. However, by identifying those marbles that are common across many marble spaces, we can identify the exposures and environments that are more critical for intervention and prevention efforts.

Public Health Implications of Disease Causation

We have shown through our marble example that each individual's marble jar or marble space may be unique, with or without overlap across individuals.

Individuals with certain combination of marbles develop specific health indicators of interest.

At the population level, epidemiologists look for the marbles that are most common across individuals with disease compared to those without and whether these marbles are shared (through infection or clustering) or they have the same marbles but are not shared (same genetic mutation, consumption of fatty food). Why? Because by removing any one of the marbles, we can prevent disease in all individuals with that marble in their jar. The more individuals for whom a certain component cause is necessary, the more disease will be prevented by removing that marble from the population.

In Figure 7.5, we show three individuals and marble jars that caused the disease in each of them. If Person 1 were not exposed to marble W, for example, Person 1 would not develop the disease. At a population level, if we prevent exposure to marble Z, Person 2 and Person 3 would not develop the disease. As public health professionals, would we focus on preventing marble W, X, Y, or Z? We would work to prevent Y, as we would get the most benefit at the population level—none of the three people would develop the disease. This illustrates a central point in public health intervention for an epidemiology of consequence: We conduct epidemiologic studies to identify those causes that render the most benefit for the largest portion of the population. This public health principle motivates many public health programs: vaccination requirements for schools, policies and laws that restrict access to unhealthy substances such as cigarettes and alcohol, and the promotion of opportunities for regular and safe exercise and availability of fresh food. These efforts target the causes that we believe to be in the marble jars of the greatest number of people who acquire common chronic diseases.

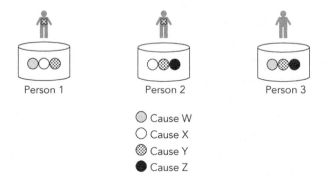

FIGURE 7.5 Exposure combinations and disease causation.

Summary

At the individual level, people acquire disease through a set of component causes that were all necessary for that individual but often alone were insufficient; at the population level, there is often no single cause that is present in all cases and no single group of causes that inevitably produce disease. Multifactorial and complex chronic diseases typically are caused by a host of factors that together contribute to the development of the disease. These are typically termed *risk factors* in the literature. These risk factors are causes of disease because they are part of at least one person's sufficient cause that resulted in the disease. By identifying those risk factors—those component causes—that are part of the marble space for the most individuals, we can have the greatest impact on reducing disease for the greatest number of people.

From Marble Space to Probability: Understanding Disease Causation in a Non-Deterministic World

We now understand that the process of disease development may begin pre-conceptually and continue until the moment that the disease occurs. Often many causes have to align for a disease to occur in an individual. Single causes are rarely sufficient alone. Causes can be shared across people or unique to a certain person. The idea that many causes must accumulate throughout the life course before the disease manifests is, in epidemiology, expressed as the concept of interaction. That is, if seven marbles are all necessary to cause disease in an individual, than all of these marbles interact with each other. By preventing exposure to even one marble, the disease will not occur from any marble.

The concept of interaction underlies all of our theories of causation for complex diseases. When component causes are unnecessary and insufficient at the population level, they will only be able to act in the presence of other causes (Rothman, 1976; Rothman & Greenland, 2005); or, in terms of our marble analogy, if single marbles are not sufficient to fill the marble jar, the disease will only occur when a specific assortment of marbles is present in the jar. Causes need not be temporally proximal to the exposure of interest; that is, one cause can occur early in life, and an interacting cause can occur late in life. In the following, we give some examples of the power of interaction as a defining concept for causal inference.

Example 1: Diet and Phenylketonuria

We begin with an example focusing on two causes of disease that interact.

Phenylketonuria (PKU) is a rare disorder present at birth characterized by the inability to process a certain amino acid, phenylalanine. The disorder, when untreated, results include mental retardation, altered appearance (light skin and hair), and seizures and hyperactivity. The necessary cause for PKU is inheriting a particular genetic sequence from both the mother and father. However, this inherited genetic sequence will not result in the expressed phenotype unless an individual eats a diet rich in phenylalanine. Therefore, a diet rich in phenylalanine is also necessary for the symptoms of PKU to manifest.

Individuals who do not possess the particular genetic sequence can consume all of the phenylalanine that they desire. Those who do posses the particular genetic sequence can avoid PKU by abstaining from foods with phenylalanine. Is genetic sequence a cause of PKU? Yes, because only individuals who have the particular genetic sequence have the potential to develop PKU. However, not everyone with the particular genetic sequence will develop PKU. Is phenylalanine in the diet a cause of the symptoms PKU? Yes, because only individuals who consume phenylalanine have the potential to develop PKU. However, not everyone who consumes phenylalanine will develop PKU. Only those with both the particular genetic sequence and phenylalanine in their diet will develop PKU.

In sum, there are two necessary causes of PKU, both of which interact to produce the expression of the disease. Neither is sufficient on its own. By interaction, we mean that only individuals who have the particular genetic sequence and consume phenylalanine will manifest PKU.

Example 2: Food Environment and Obesity

Now we move to an example focusing on many causes of disease.

The worldwide epidemic of obesity continues to move to the forefront of global public health priorities. Obesity is a complex health outcome with causes throughout the life course. For example, there is considerable interest in identifying genetic variants that are involved in the process of increasing and maintaining high weight (Bell, Walley, & Froguel, 2005). Furthermore, the impact of the in utero environment on obesity in childhood and adulthood has long been of interest. Familial factors in childhood such as food insecurity and socioeconomic position as well as contextual factors such as availability of healthy food and food cost are also implicated in the obesity epidemic (Adams, Grummer-Strawn, & Chavez, 2003). Among both children and adults, health behaviors are also central causes of obesity. Individuals who consume high-sugar, low-nutrient foods such as sugar-sweetened beverages (SSBs) are at high risk for weight gain and potentially obesity. However, consumption of SSBs alone is not sufficient to cause obesity. The combination of high SSB consumption, low amounts of physical activity, and perhaps genetic predisposition that regulates the body's ability to metabolize sugar may all work together to cause obesity in some people. In others, obesity may result from metabolic patterns resulting from intrauterine growth restriction, a diet of inexpensive fatty food during childhood, and stressful life experiences. Given that there is no single sufficient or necessary cause of obesity, understanding obesity requires us to conceptualize many diverse causes interacting together to result in each obesity case.

Epidemiology and Probability

These examples make clear why epidemiology is probabilistic rather than deterministic. The reason why we frequently say that many exposures that we study "increase the risk of" rather than "always cause" disease in populations is that most of the time we are considering causes that are, at the individual level, insufficient without other causes. Also, we can rarely identify the myriad of the component causes in all of the marble jars that will work together to cause disease.

The probabilistic nature of epidemiologic causes may be best understood through a simple hypothetical example. Suppose that disease A is caused by the interaction of X, Y, and Z. Put another way, X, Y, and Z are causes of disease A. None of them is sufficient alone to cause A, but all of them together are sufficient to cause A. The reader might say, "Why do we not just measure X, Y, and Z in everyone?" In reality, we often do not have the opportunity to measure all the potential component causes or to map out which ones interact in different individuals.

In a population of 100 people, the only people who will get the disease are those exposed to all three X, Y, and Z causes. Thus, 100% of the people exposed to X, Y, and Z get the disease; whereas 0% of people with any other combination of exposure will get the disease. We can determine with 100%

Table 7.2 Hypothetical Example Where X, Y, and Z Are Component Causes and All Are Measured

	Exposure			
	X	Y	Z	
Number of people with this interaction				Probability of disease
10	☑	☑	☑	100%
8	☑		☑	0%
11	☑	☑		0%
5		☑	☑	0%
9	☑			0%
3		☑		0%
12			☑	0%
42				0%

certainty who will develop the disease and who will not if we know whether they are exposed to X, Y, and Z.

Given the preceding, if we had knowledge of every individual's exposure to X, Y, and Z, we would be able to fully determine who will develop the disease and who will not. Those who are exposed to all three factors will develop the disease, and no other individuals will develop the disease.

Suppose, however, that we have only measured exposure X and do not have knowledge of Y and Z. From Table 7.2, counting the individuals who are exposed to X, regardless of Y and Z exposures, we get 38 (10 + 8 + 11 + 9). Of those 38, 10 have the disease (those who are also exposed to Y and Z). The prevalence of disease given exposure to X is

$$P\left(D|\text{exposed to X}\right) = \frac{10}{38} = 0.26$$

The probability of disease given exposure to X is 26%. If we knew whether an individual was also exposed to Y and Z, we could provide more information than the single probability. In fact, if we had knowledge of Y and Z, we could fully determine who has the disease. But we do not have knowledge of Y and Z; therefore, we have now have moved from deterministic to probabilistic, which is at heart what we do in all of epidemiology. One way to conceptualize this distinction between deterministic and probabilistic is based on whether we have the whole picture or part of the picture. If we do not know all of the exposures that are involved in producing a particular outcome (which is almost always the case), the best we can do is make a probability statement that quantifies the risk of developing the disease when we know of exposure to X but have no information on other exposures.

This simple example can be generalized to the broader field of epidemiology when we examine the potential causes of disease. We examine whether a factor increases the risk for disease because we believe that factor to be a cause that acts in concert with many other causes. In theory, if we had knowledge of all causes, we could move beyond statements about increasing risk to develop fully deterministic models. However, in practice, this is likely impossible, especially given that stochastic (unpredictable) factors also play a role in each individual's disease occurrence (Davey Smith, 2011).

In our simple example, there was only one way to get disease: exposure to X, Y, and Z. In reality, there are likely many ways to get the disease. We therefore provide a more complicated example (yet still likely simplistic in the context of real life disease) of the relation between deterministic and probabilistic epidemiology in Box 7.3 of the online material that accompanies this chapter in which we have two sufficient causes that produce disease.

Summary: From the Unobservable to the Observed— Causal Architecture in the Real World

The counterfactual can never be observed. We cannot hold everything in the world—including time—constant and observe an individual under two conditions simultaneously. The marbles and marble jars can never be observed. All that was described in this chapter is the predominant theory for the causal architecture that underlies human health, which is unseen, but from which we can more rigorously form theories and hypotheses and learn from the data that we can observe. Thus, the counterfactual framework is one that is useful for thinking about the definition of a causal effect, but it is not a practical solution for evaluating whether epidemiologic evidence is consistent with a causal effect of an exposure on a health outcome.

We decide whether an exposure is a cause of adverse health by weighing the totality of epidemiologic evidence. Usually, no single study is sufficient to prove whether an exposure is a cause of a health indicator. We triangulate multiple forms of evidence, from animal studies to human studies, and we construct rigorous comparisons across multiple study designs that put our causal hypotheses to the test. The process of causal inference in practice is typically based on a progression of evidence, sifting through multiple different methodological and analytic issues across many studies and designs to form a reasoned conclusion.

In the next chapters, we describe how to design and analyze epidemiologic studies to optimize the validity of our results. The goal of these studies is to generate a body of literature that allows us to form consensus about the strength of the evidence for or against a particular exposure or set of exposures as causally related to a health outcome of interest.

References

Adams, E. J., Grummer-Strawn, L., & Chavez, G. (2003). Food insecurity is associated with increased risk of obesity in California women. *Journal of Nutrition, 133,* 1070–1074.

Bell, C. G., Walley, A. J., & Froguel, P. (2005). The genetics of human obesity. *Nature Reviews Genetics, 6,* 221–234.

Christakis, N. A., & Fowler, J. H. (2007). The spread of obesity in a large social network over 32 years. *New England Journal of Medicine, 357,* 370–379.

Davey Smith, G. (2011). Epidemiology, epigenetics and the "Gloomy Prospect": Embracing randomness in population health research and practice. *International Journal of Epidemiology, 40,* 537–562.

Galea, S., Nandi, A., & Vlahov, D. (2004). The social epidemiology of substance use. *Epidemiologic Reviews, 26,* 36–52.

Lumey, L. H., Stein, A. D., & Susser, E. (2011). Prenatal famine and adult health. *Annual Review of Public Health, 32,* 237–262.

Kramer, M. S. (1987). Determinants of low birth weight: Methodological assessment and meta-analysis. *Bulletin of the World Health Organization, 65,* 663–737.

Krug, E. G., Mercy, J. A., Dahlberg, L. L., & Zwi, A. B. (2002). The world report on violence and health. *Lancet, 360*(9339), 1083–1088.

Rothman, K. J. (1976). Causes. *American Journal of Epidemiology, 104,* 587–592.

Rothman, K. J. (2008). Causation and Causal Inference. In K. J. Rothman, S. Greenland, & T. L. Lash (Eds.), *Modern Epidemiology* (3rd ed., pp. 5–31). Philadelphia: Lippincott Williams & Wilkins.

Rothman, K. J., & Greenland, S. (2005). Causation and causal inference in epidemiology. *American Journal of Public Health, 95*(S1), S144–S150.

Schwartz, S., & Susser, E. (2006). What is a cause? In E. Susser, S. M. Schwartz, A. Morabia, & E. Bromet (Eds.), *Psychiatric epidemiology: Searching for the causes of mental disorders* (pp. 33–42). New York: Oxford University Press.

Urberg, K. A., Shyu, S. J., & Liang, J. (1990). Peer influence in adolescent cigarette smoking. *Addictive Behaviors, 15,* 247–255.

Walters, K., Breeze, E., Wilkinson, P., Price, G. M., Bulpitt, C. J., & Fletcher, A. (2004). Local area deprivation and urban-rural differences in anxiety and depression among people older than 75 years in Britain. *American Journal of Public Health, 94,* 1768–1774.

Zuber, J. (2012). Healthcare for the undocumented: Solving a public health crisis in the U.S. *Journal of Contemporary Health Law and Policy, 28,* 350–380.

8

Is the Association Causal, or Are There Alternative Explanations?

WE DISCUSSED IN Chapter 7 how to conceptualize an exposure as a potential cause of disease within the counterfactual framework: Would the disease have occurred when and how it did without the exposure, or without the amount of exposure that occurred, the timing of exposure, or within the context of multiple exposures? These counterfactual questions have become foundational to most causal thinking in epidemiology. However, they are conceptual questions that cannot be empirically answered in our data. When we conduct epidemiologic studies and derive associations between exposures and health outcomes, a new question emerges: Does the association that we measure in our data reflect the amount of excess disease that occurred due to the effects of the exposure (i.e., would the risk of disease have been different if those who were exposed had not been exposed), or could there be alternative explanations for the study findings other than a causal explanation? This is a much more difficult question to answer and often requires triangulation of evidence from multiple studies with various designs to answer.

This leads us to further into Step 5 of our seven-step approach to conducting an epidemiologic study. Specifically, once we identify a population, take a sample of that population, count the cases of adverse health, and compare health indicators across exposure categories, we need to decide whether our results reflect causal associations. To answer the question of whether the associations observed in our data from a single study reflect causal associations, we need to engage in thought experiments about the distributions of causes of health indicators other than the hypothesized exposure and how comparable those exposed and unexposed in the study sample are on these hypothesized alternative causes.

The idea of comparability of exposed and unexposed groups is at the heart of all epidemiologic inferential thinking and needs to be mastered to address questions about whether a particular exposure is the cause of a particular health indicator or whether an observed association is explained by alternative explanations. In this chapter, we guide the reader through logical steps to illustrate what we mean by comparability and why it matters.

When Does an Exposure Cause a Health Indicator? It All Starts With the Individual

Our counterfactual definition specifies that a cause of a health indicator is one for which the health indicator would not have occurred when and how it did in the absence of the exposure. For this exposition, we assume that the health indicator is a disease. The ideal experiment in which to observe whether the disease would have occurred would be to take the same person observed over the same time period, once with the exposure and once without the exposure. All other characteristics of the person, place, and time are held constant; the only factor that changes is the exposure. While of course we cannot observe the same person at the same exact time under a condition of exposure and simultaneously under a condition of no exposure, we can engage in the thought experiment of observing the same individual under simultaneous conditions. If the disease occurs when the exposure is present but not when the exposure is absent, we can say with assurance that the exposure is causal for that individual (likewise, if we are studying a hypothetical protective exposure, we would say it is causal if the disease does not occur when the exposure is present but does occur in the absence of exposure). This situation is shown in Person 1 of Figure 8.1. Person 1 has the disease when exposed. If we

Person 1 observed at the same time
(once with the exposure and once
without the exposure)

Person 2 observed at the same time
(once with the exposure and once
without the exposure)

FIGURE 8.1 Observing individuals under simultaneous conditions.

were able to observe the same person at the same time without the exposure, she would not have the disease. Thus, the exposure is causal for that person. Person 2 also has the disease when exposed. If we were able to observe the same person at the same time without the exposure, however, she would still have the disease. Thus, the exposure is not causal for Person 2.

Other Causes of the Outcome Complicate Causal Inference: The Introduction of Dots

Why would an exposure be causal for Person 1 but not causal for Person 2? To understand why, remember that there may be many causes of a particular health outcome. For example, in Chapter 7 we provided a hypothetical example of factors that cause diabetes. We saw that some people acquired diabetes through some combination of exposures that included lack of preventive care, whereas others acquired diabetes through some combination of exposures that included family history of diabetes. Thus, individuals can be exposed to a variable of interest and also experience the health outcome, but the exposure will not have been the cause of their disease. For example, consider the following scenario.

Disease X has two sufficient causes (or marble jars): exposure to A, B, and C or exposure to E, F, and G. An individual is exposed to A, B, C, E, and G. This individual will get the disease because she is exposed to A, B, and C. She is also exposed to E; however, exposure to E is not causal for this individual because she does not have all of the other exposures that fill the marble jar with E. Thus, individual A is exposed to E, has the disease, but E is not causal for this individual.

If we are interested in whether exposure to E causes the disease, we can consider A, B, and C as other causes of the disease that are in a different marble jar than the exposure of interest. Individuals with any of the hypothesized component causes of the outcome (A, B, or C) that are not in a marble jar with exposure (E) we now denote with dots as a way to demarcate other causes of disease aside from the exposure of interest. Individuals possessing a full marble jar of component causes to produce the outcome will develop the disease whether exposed or not; thus, the exposure is not causal for these individuals.

Now, we return to Person 1 and Person 2 from Figure 8.1. Shown in Figure 8.2 are these individuals again, and again they are observed under two exposure conditions (exposed and unexposed) simultaneously. Person 1 does not have dots, indicating that this person is not exposed to other causes of

Person 1 observed at the same time
(once with the exposure and once
without the exposure)

Person 2 observed at the same time
(once with the exposure and once
without the exposure)

FIGURE 8.2 Observing individuals under simultaneous conditions with multiple causes.

disease outside of the exposure of interest and the component causes that are in a marble jar with that exposure. Again, the exposure for this person was causal because they have the disease when exposed and they do not have the disease when not exposed. For Person 2, we can now see why the person had the disease regardless of exposure. Person 2 had a marble jar of component causes sufficient to produce the disease (e.g., in our example, she was exposed to A, B, and C), and this marble jar did not include the exposure of interest. Thus, this person was going to get the disease whether exposed or not. It is these other causes of disease—those that are not in a sufficient cause with the exposure of interest—that complicate causal inference. If we know about the other causes of disease, we can mitigate their effects through study design or analysis. If we do not know about the other causes of disease, we may make incorrect causal inferences based on our measures of association from epidemiologic studies.

Moving From the Individual to the Comparison of Groups

In epidemiologic studies, we example groups of exposed and unexposed people rather than an individual exposed or unexposed person. However, the concepts described previously remain applicable: If we could observe the same group of people over the same time period but remove the exposure, the causal effect of the exposure is the difference in the number of cases that occur with the exposure and the number of cases that occur without the exposure. Consider the sample of individuals shown in Figure 8.3. When we observe these 10 people, all of whom are exposed, we see that 5 develop the disease. If we were able to observe all 10 people without the exposure, holding

Ten people, all exposed

The same ten people observed at the
same time without the exposure

FIGURE 8.3 Observing a group of individuals under simultaneous conditions.

all else constant, we see that 3 would develop the disease. Thus, there were 2 excess cases of disease that were due to the causal effect of the exposure on the outcome.

Given that there were 5 cases of disease in the exposed group, why are there only 2 excess cases of disease due to the exposure? We return to the concept of dots, individuals who are exposed to an alternative cause of disease, and in fact may have a collection of component causes that produce the disease that does not include the exposure. In Figure 8.4 we show the same set of 10 people, but we have now added dots. These dots denote people who have another cause of disease outside of the exposure. They may or may not have the causal partners of this alternative cause to fill the marble jar; thus, only a portion of the individuals with dots will evince the disease.

Ten people, all exposed

The same ten people observed at the
same time without the exposure

FIGURE 8.4 Observing a group of individuals under simultaneous conditions with multiple causes.

We see that among the 5 individuals who became diseased when exposed, 3 had dots and 2 did not have dots. We also see that 2 people who did not become diseased had dots. If we were able to observe the same 10 people under the condition of no exposure, we see that 3 people with dots still become diseased—thus the exposure was not causal for those individuals. Considering the 2 people who have dots but do not become diseased, note that the dots denote only that these individuals are exposed to an alternative cause; they may not possess all of the component causes to fill a marble jar. Overall, we now see that there are 2 excess cases of disease that are due to exposure because, among the 5 exposed individuals who develop the disease, 3 would have developed the disease even in the absence of exposure due to the presence of a set of alternative causes that are sufficient.

From Comparison of Groups to Epidemiologic Study: The Importance of Comparability

We cannot observe the same people over the same period with and without exposure; we cannot hold time constant and we cannot magically change individuals from exposed to unexposed (or vice versa). Instead, we can compare groups of exposed and unexposed people, often observed in parallel over the same time period. As a core principle of epidemiologic methods, we take an exposed group of people and compare risk or prevalence of health outcomes to a group of unexposed people. However, when we engage in this group comparison, we must know how comparable these two groups are to each other in terms of the number of individuals with dots (i.e., causes of the disease other than the exposure of interest and not in the same marble jar as the exposure of interest).

Remember that in Figure 8.4 we were able to determine that there were two excess cases of disease due to exposure because out of the five cases who got the disease when exposed, three would have gotten the disease even if they had not been exposed. These two groups were perfectly comparable— they were the same people observed with and without exposure at the same place and time. In reality, we can never compare the fact to the counterfactual (Rubin, 1974). The best we can do in an epidemiologic study is to choose an unexposed group to be so similar to the exposed group that it represents the experience of the exposed group had they not been exposed. In other words, we need the exposed and unexposed to be comparable. By comparable, we mean "how close is the unexposed group to what I would expect the exposed group to resemble if they were not exposed?"

To answer this question, we need to know about the distribution of other causes of disease, those causes that are not in the marble jar of the exposure of interest, between the exposed and unexposed groups. In other words, we need to know how many individuals have dots in the exposed and unexposed groups. Consider two hypothetical epidemiologic studies in which we are comparing a group of exposed individuals to a set of different individuals who are unexposed. In this example, there is one additional way to get the disease that does not include the exposure: this is through a pathway that contains a different exposure that we denote with dots. In our hypothetical example, we can perfectly measure exposure, disease, and the presence of the alternative exposure denoted with dots.

We estimate the risk of disease given exposure and compare it to the risk of disease given no exposure. Figure 8.5 shows the data from Study 1. Assume that each person in the figure represents data for 10 people. Thus, there are 10 people in the figure who are exposed, and these represent 100 exposed persons; 6 of the exposed are diseased, and they represent 60 exposed persons. Similarly, 10 people in the figure are unexposed, representing 100 unexposed persons, and 3 have the disease, representing 30 diseased persons.

The risk of disease is 2.0 times higher in the exposed compared to the unexposed, and there are 30 excess cases of disease per 100 exposed. Are these 30 excess cases of disease due to the exposure? To answer this question, we look at the distribution of dots. We see that 7 of the 100 individuals have dots, both

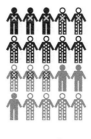

$$\text{Risk Ratio:} \frac{\frac{60}{100}}{\frac{30}{100}} = 2.0$$

$$\text{Risk difference:} \left(\frac{60}{100}\right) - \left(\frac{30}{100}\right) = 0.30$$

FIGURE 8.5 Epidemiologic Study 1.

in the exposed and the unexposed group. Thus, there is an even distribution of dots across exposure conditions, and all 30 excess cases are attributable to the exposure indicating that these groups are comparable.

Now we turn to Epidemiologic Study 2. Again, each person in Figure 8.6 represents the experience of 10 people. Among the 100 exposed, the same 60 people become diseased. Among the unexposed, however, only 10 people develop the disease.

In this sample, the risk of disease is 6.0 times higher in the exposed compared to the unexposed, and there are 50 excess cases of disease per 100 exposed. Are these excess cases of disease due to the exposure? We turn to the distribution of dots in the exposed and in the unexposed. Among the exposed, there are 70 individuals with dots. Among the unexposed, however, there are only 30 with dots. Thus, there is an unequal distribution of other causes of disease between the exposed and the unexposed. Dots are more common in the exposed than in the unexposed. These exposure groups are not comparable. We would obtain an incorrect causal inference, concluding that exposure is responsible for more cases of disease than it actually is, by relying on Epidemiologic Study 2.

In epidemiology, factors that contribute to non-comparability between exposed and unexposed are often termed *confounders,* and the magnitude of the difference between the observed association and the true association is often called the *amount of confounding.* Thus, a synonymous term for non-comparability is *confounding.*

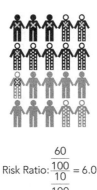

$$\text{Risk Ratio:} \frac{\frac{60}{100}}{\frac{10}{100}} = 6.0$$

$$\text{Risk difference:} \left(\frac{60}{100}\right) - \left(\frac{10}{100}\right) = 50$$

FIGURE 8.6 Epidemiologic Study 2.

Summary

Ideally, to understand whether an exposure actually causes an outcome, we would observe an individual or group of individuals under two conditions simultaneously: exposed and unexposed. If we could do this, we would conclude that an exposure is responsible for disease if an individual becomes diseased when exposed but not when unexposed. This is impossible, however, so we compare two groups of people: one group that is exposed and a different group that is unexposed. We are still be able to estimate the excess cases of disease due to the exposure as long as the distribution of other causes that are not in the marble jar of the exposure of interest of disease is equal between the groups. In other words, the two groups should be comparable with respect to all other causes of disease, with the only difference between the two groups being the exposure of interest. Throughout the history of epidemiology, there have been many circumstances in which data have led to spurious findings because of non-comparability (see Box 8.1, "Hormone Replacement Therapy: A Cautionary Tale" in the online material that accompanies Chapter 8). Careful assessment and control of these sources of non-comparability, either in the design or analysis phase of the study, is one of the most important roles of the epidemiologist in the health sciences.

Now that we understand that causal inference from our study sample will not be accurate if other causes of disease are not equally distributed between exposed and unexposed groups, the natural question is how this non-comparability arises in actual epidemiologic studies and what we can do about it. In the next chapter, we detail the four common ways in which non-comparability arises in epidemiologic studies. In Chapter 10, we discuss strategies for mitigating non-comparability in the design of the study and analysis of the study data.

Reference

Rubin, D. B. (1974). Estimating causal effects of treatments in randomized and nonrandomized studies. *Journal of Educational Psychology, 56*, 688–701.

9

How Do Noncausal Associations Arise?

WE REMAIN FOCUSED in this chapter on Step 5 of our seven-step guide to epidemiologic studies, which is rigorously assessing whether the associations observed in our data reflect causal effects of exposures on health indicators. In Chapter 8, we described how non-comparability between exposed and unexposed on other causes of health indicators is at the root of many noncausal associations in epidemiologic studies. In this chapter, we describe four ways in which non-comparability between exposed and unexposed groups in an epidemiologic study can arise: (a) because of chance in the sampling process, (b) because of associated causes, (c) because of improper selection of study subjects or loss to follow-up, and (d) because of misclassification of exposure and disease status.

Sources of Non-Comparability: Random Chance

In Chapter 4, we discussed variability when taking a sample of the population. By chance alone, the sample that we collect may have an unequal distribution of other causes of the health indicator of interest. We use confidence intervals around our measures of association to put bounds around a range of associations that reflect these possible unequal distributions due to chance in the sampling process. However, this confidence interval does not tell us how likely the estimate is to be causal with any certainty because it only accounts for chance in unequally distributing causes of disease, other than the hypothesized exposure of interest, between groups. There may be, and likely will be, non-chance reasons why other causes of disease are unequally distributed across groups. The possibility of non-comparability arising from random chance process decreases by increasing the sample size and the precision of the measures. At the extreme, if we were able to interview the whole population, for example, random chance in the sampling process would have no effect on our estimates. However, even if we study the whole population, we still may not obtain a causal effect of the exposure on the outcome because of the other ways in which non-comparability can arise.

Sources of Non-Comparability: Associated Causes

Non-comparability can arise between two or more groups simply because these groups are different from each other in multiple ways that affect health. For example, people who eat a lot of leafy green vegetables every day may be more likely to exercise, less likely to smoke or use illicit substances, and generally more health conscious than individuals who eat few leafy green vegetables every day. If we endeavor to know whether leafy green vegetable consumption is good for health, we must recognize these group differences and account for them in our epidemiologic study design and analysis. These differences across exposed and unexposed groups are often termed confounders in epidemiology; more generally, a confounder is a variable that contributes to non-comparability between the exposed and unexposed. The fact that people select their own health behaviors inevitably means that causes of adverse health will be associated with each other: People who engage in one particular potentially problematic health behavior are more likely to engage in more than one compared to people who do not engage in that health behavior. Thus, when we observe people over time attempting to document an association between a hypothesized exposure and outcome, we must consider what causes of the outcome may travel with the hypothesized exposure and account for these traveling partners in our epidemiologic design and analysis.

Example: Alcohol Consumption and Risk of Esophageal Cancer

Chronic heavy alcohol consumption is associated with numerous adverse health outcomes—but how much of the association is due to the effects of alcohol versus the effects of other factors?

Population-based studies indicate that chronic heavy drinkers have about 4 times the risk of developing esophageal cancer compared to non-heavy drinkers (Blot, 1992; Franceschi et al., 1990). If causal, this evidence indicates that public health recommendations should focus on reducing heavy alcohol

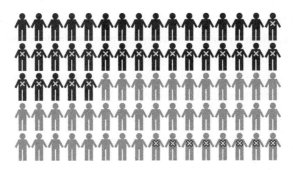

FIGURE 9.1 Sample for study of esophageal cancer in heavy drinkers and non-heavy drinkers.

consumption in the population. As a heuristic example, we understand how this could potentially be a noncausal association in our data.

We define the population of interest as men over the age of 50 in Farrlandia. For the example, we collect a sample of 800 men. None of the 800 men have esophageal cancer at the start of the study, and we follow them for 20 years with no loss to follow-up. Of these 800, 370 are heavy drinkers and 430 are not. Of the 370 heavy drinkers, 220 develop esophageal cancer. Of the 430 non-heavy drinkers, 80 develop esophageal cancer. Shown in Figure 9.1 is the sample of men from Farrlandia, with each person in the figure representing the experience of 10 members of our sample.

Given that there was no loss to follow-up in our study, the conditional risk of disease in the exposed and unexposed are appropriate measures for comparison. The data from the study are presented in Figure 9.2.

Thus, in our sample, heavy drinkers have 3.20 times the risk of developing esophageal cancer over 20 years compared with non-heavy drinkers (see Figure 9.2). Further, there is an excess of 40 cases of esophageal cancer for every 100 individuals followed for 20 years associated with heavy alcohol consumption. But how do we know the excess in cancer among drinkers is caused by their alcohol consumption?

Individuals who consume heavy amounts of alcohol and individuals who do not are likely very different groups of people. We know that heavy alcohol consumers are more likely to be men than women, for example (Hasin, Stinson, Ogburn, & Grant, 2007). Moderate alcohol consumers also watch other aspects of their diet more carefully, consuming more fresh fruits and vegetables and less saturated fat (Connor, 2006). When we observe that heavy alcohol consumers are more likely to develop an adverse health outcome than other groups, then we do not know whether it was the heavy

	Health indicator present	Health indicator absent	**Total**
Exposed	220	150	370
Unexposed	80	350	430
Total	300	500	800

$$P(D \mid E+) = \frac{220}{370} = 0.59$$

$$P(D \mid E-) = \frac{80}{430} = 0.19$$

$$\text{Risk ratio} = \frac{0.59}{0.19} = 3.20[95\% \text{ CI } (2.58, 3.96)]$$

$$\text{Risk difference} = 0.59 - 0.19 = 0.41[95\% \text{ CI}(0.35, 0.47)]$$

FIGURE 9.2 Association between heavy drinking and esophageal cancer.

alcohol consumption that caused the adverse health outcome or one of the other factors that is associated with heavy alcohol consumption.

We consider one specific factor that we know differs between individuals who consume heavy amounts of alcohol and those who do not: cigarette smoking.[1] Cigarette smoking is in and of itself a potential cause of esophageal cancer (Choi & Kahyo, 1991), and we would expect that a group of heavy drinkers would have a higher proportion of smokers. Therefore, could the smokers be driving the observed association with esophageal cancer?

To examine this, in Figure 9.3, we return to the graphical representation of dots in our samples from Farrlandia. Remember from Chapter 8 that we used dots to denote individuals who were exposed to potential causes of disease other than the main exposure of interest.

Among the 370 heavy drinkers, 310 have dots—thus 310 are smokers, or 83.8%. Among the 430 non-heavy drinkers, 270 have dots—thus 270 are smokers, or 62.8%. We can confirm in our data, then, that smoking is more common among the heavy drinkers: 83.8% versus 62.8%.

Next, we need to determine whether the smokers are more likely to develop esophageal cancer than non-smokers, regardless of whether they are heavy drinkers. To examine this, we create a 2 × 2 table; instead of black and grey

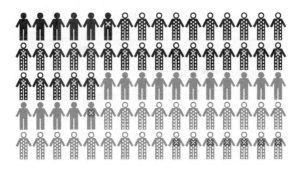

FIGURE 9.3 Source of non-comparability: smoking and esophageal cancer.

denoting exposed and unexposed, now we ignore color and focus on dots or no dots. The data from the study are presented in Figure 9.4.

The total number with dots is 580 (310 of the heavy drinkers and 270 of the non-heavy drinkers). Among these 580, 280 have esophageal cancer, yielding a conditional probability of cancer among the smokers of 48.3%. The total number without dots is 320. Among these, 20 have cancer, yielding a conditional probability of cancer among the non-smokers of 6.3%. We can confirm in our data, then, that smoking is associated with esophageal cancer in these data.

Thus, smoking is a source of non-comparability in our data, and the effects of smoking on esophageal cancer will obscure our assessment of the effects of heavy alcohol consumption on esophageal cancer. Smoking is a confounder of this association. We detail ways in which to mitigate the effects of these confounding variables in the design and analysis of the study in Chapter 10.

	Health indicator present		Health indicator absent		**Total**
Exposed (Dots)	210	+ 70 = 280	100	+ 200 = 300	580
Unexposed (Dots)	10	+ 10 = 20	150	+ 150 = 300	320
Total	300		600		900

FIGURE 9.4 Association between smoking and esophageal cancer.

Sources of Non-Comparability: Selection and Follow-Up of Study Subjects

In Chapter 4, we described three foundational ways in which to take a representative or purposive sample from a dynamically changing population to conduct an epidemiologic study: (a) we can select a sample at a particular point in time, (b) we can select a sample of disease-free individuals and follow them forward in time, or (c) we can select a certain number of cases and non-cases and examine exposure histories. Regardless of the study design, which dictates when the sample is selected from a dynamic underlying population, the same issue arises when we are trying to estimate whether a hypothesized exposure is a cause of an outcome: Are the exposed and unexposed comparable with respect to all causes of disease other than the exposure? In the following, we discuss various scenarios in which non-comparability between exposed and unexposed can arise in basic epidemiologic study designs.

Non-Comparability When a Sample Is Followed Forward in Time

Non-comparability can arise in two main ways when following individuals forward in time. First, we might select exposed and unexposed in such a way that there is non-comparability between groups at baseline. Second, non-comparability can arise if there is loss to follow-up over time that is associated with both exposure and health indicator status. We provide a quantitative example of each to illustrate principles of non-comparability due to selection and follow-up.

Non-Comparability When a Sample Is Initially Selected at Baseline

As we have detailed, non-comparability arises when exposed and unexposed groups have different distributions of other causes of health indicators apart from the exposure of interest. The principle applies when considering the selection of individuals into the study for prospective follow-up. For example, if eligibility criteria, recruitment, or participation differ between exposed and unexposed, the result may be that the exposed and unexposed groups in the sample are not comparable on all causes of the health indicator other than the exposure of interest.

As an example, we conduct a study of pesticide exposure and incidence of lung cancer. The exposed group is drawn from farm workers who work frequently with pesticides. For an unexposed group, we place advertisements in the communities around the farms looking for individuals free of lung cancer who have never worked with pesticides and are interested in participating in a study about lung cancer. The advertisement notes free regular screening and medical care for those who agree to participate. Most people who sign up from the advertisements to be a part of the unexposed group either smoke or have a family history of lung cancer because they are worried about their health and interested in the medical services provided. Will the unexposed group be comparable with the exposed group?

The unexposed group has a higher proportion of smokers and individuals with potential genetic predisposition to lung cancer compared with the exposed. Therefore, the risk of lung cancer is likely going to be higher in the unexposed group selected for the study than in the counterfactual of the farm workers (i.e., the farm workers' risk of lung cancer group if they had not been exposed to pesticides). Any causal effect of pesticide exposure on lung cancer will be underestimated in this study. We show the effect of this non-comparability quantitatively in Box 9.1 of the online material that accompanies this chapter.

Non-Comparability Arising During Follow-Up of Study Subjects

When we follow a group of disease-free individuals forward in time to estimate differences in risk across exposure groups, non-comparability can arise if a different proportion of individuals who eventually develop the disease drop out of the study compared with people who do not eventually develop the disease. Because they drop out, however, we as investigators never know whether they eventually develop the disease. Thus, non-comparability due to loss to follow-up cannot be empirically evaluated. However, it is still critical to consider whether loss to follow-up in an epidemiologic sample could potentially be associated with the study outcome and consider the ways in which this association may affect study estimates.

We demonstrate the potentially biasing effects of loss to follow-up with the example research question of the association between drug education and subsequent illicit drug use. We conduct a study of the long-term effect of an illicit drug education program in high school on incident drug use in adulthood. Students in high schools either received the drug education program or did not, and these students were followed into adulthood and surveyed every 2 years regarding first use of illicit drugs. There is substantial loss to follow-up in both groups, those who received drug education and those who did not, and we are concerned that individuals who eventually used drugs were more likely to drop out than individuals who did not use drugs. By the end of the study, will the unexposed group be non-comparable with the exposed group? What if this dropping out is also related to whether they had drug education in high school?

The health indicator of interest in the study is first use of an illicit drug. The exposure, for our purposes, will be the absence of drug education during high school. We hypothesize that individuals who did not have drug education in high school are at increased risk for illicit drug use into adulthood compared with individuals who did receive drug education. The true association in our Farrlandia sample without any loss to follow-up is in Figure 9.5, which represents what we would have observed if we had been able to observe all individuals in the study sample for four time points (each time point being 2 years apart, for a total of 6 years). Each person in the figure represents the experience of 10 people in our sample.

In the sample with no loss to follow-up, we observe that individuals without drug education have 2.0 times the risk, 2.17 times the rate, and 2.67 times the odds of incident illicit drug use over 6 years compared with individuals who did have drug education. We expect 20 excess illicit drug users per 100 persons over 6 years who do not receive drug education in high school, and 4.2 cases per 100 person years of exposure associated with lack of drug education.

LOSS TO FOLLOW-UP THAT DIFFERS BY OUTCOME STATUS AND EXPOSURE STATUS

Loss to follow-up can be associated with exposure status (e.g., those who are exposed are more likely to drop out), health indicator status (e.g., those who eventually develop the health indicator are more likely to drop out), or both. In Boxes 9.2 and 9.3 of the online material that accompanies Chapter 9, we provide quantitative examples of loss to follow-up that is associated with exposure or health indicator status but not both. We focus now on the situation in which loss to follow-up is associated with exposure and health indicator status.

In our study of drug education and illicit drug use, the participants who did not receive drug education may be more likely to drop out, especially those who will eventually be illicit drug users. Thus, we have dropping out by exposure status (those who do not receive drug education are more likely to drop out); and we have dropping out by disease status (those who eventually use illicit drugs are more likely to drop out). Suppose in our study that 25% of people who never use illicit drugs drop out, and 25% of those who eventually use illicit drugs but received drug education drop out, while 50% of those who

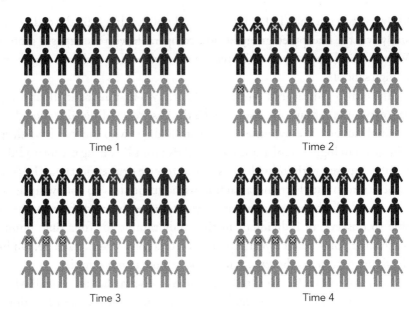

	Health indicator present	Health indicator absent	Total N	Person years
Exposed	80	120	200	1020
Unexposed	40	160	200	1120
Total N	120	280	400	2140

2x2 for Time 4

$$P(D\mid E+)=\frac{80}{200}=0.40$$

$$P(D\mid E-)=\frac{40}{200}=0.20$$

$$\text{Risk ratio}=\frac{0.40}{0.20}=2.0[95\%\ CI\ (1.45,2.77)]$$

$$\text{Risk difference}=0.40-0.20=0.20[95\%\ CI(0.11,0.29)]$$

$$\text{Rate of disease among exposed}=\frac{80}{1020}=0.078$$

FIGURE 9.5 The association between drug education and illicit drug use without any loss to follow-up.

$$\text{Rate of disease among unexposed} = \frac{40}{1120} = 0.036$$

$$\text{Rate ratio} = \frac{0.078}{0.036} = 2.17[95\% \text{ CI } (1.50, 3.21)]$$

$$\text{Rate difference} = 0.078 - 0.036 = 0.042[95\% \text{ CI}(0.02, 0.06)]$$

$$\text{Odds ratio} = \frac{\dfrac{\dfrac{80}{120}}{\dfrac{40}{120}}}{\dfrac{\dfrac{120}{280}}{\dfrac{160}{280}}} = \frac{80 * 160}{120 * 40} = 2.67 \ [95\% \text{ CI } (1.70, 4.17)]$$

FIGURE 9.5 Continued

both did not receive drug education and eventually used illicit drugs drop out. See Figure 9.6.

When more eventual illicit drug users who did not receive drug education drop out of the sample than other groups, we underestimate all measures of association, including the risk ratio, rate ratio, risk difference, and odds ratio. In general, loss to follow-up that is associated with both exposure and disease will bias all measures of association in any study design where individuals are being followed over time because non-comparability between the exposed and unexposed is introduced into the study estimates.

Whereas in this example, the resulting bias was that we underestimated the effect of drug education, there are many situations in which loss to follow-up may overestimate measures of association. For example, in a randomized clinical trial of a new drug, those who are randomized to receive the active drug and who are experiencing positive outcomes of the drug may be more likely to stay in the trial than individuals who are randomized to the drug but do not experience an improvement in symptoms. Such non-comparability would render effect estimates that are larger than the true causal estimate of the effect of the drug.

Given that we have loss to follow-up in the forthcoming examples, an appropriate measure of association between exposure and the health indicator is the rate ratio. In Box 9.4 of the online material that accompanies Chapter 9, we provide a more detailed overview of how the rate ratio for this example

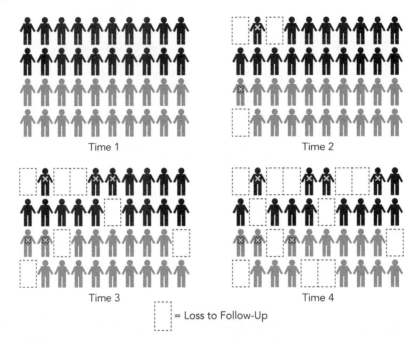

Time 1   Time 2

Time 3   Time 4

= Loss to Follow-Up

2x2 table for study participants at Time 4: Loss to follow-up by exposure and outcome status

	Health indicator present	Health indicator absent	**Total**	Person years
Exposed	40	130	170	700
Unexposed	30	120	150	920
Total	70	250	320	1620

$$P(D|E+) = \frac{40}{170} = 0.24$$

$$P(D|E-) = \frac{30}{150} = 0.20$$

$$\text{Risk ratio} = \frac{0.24}{0.20} = 1.18 \ [95\% \ CI \ (0.77, 1.79)]$$

$$\text{Risk difference} = 0.24 - 0.20 = 0.04 \ [95\% \ CI \ (-0.06, 0.13)]$$

FIGURE 9.6 Loss to follow-up by exposure and outcome status.

$$\text{Risk ratio} = \frac{0.24}{0.20} = 1.18 \; [95\% \; \text{CI} \; (0.77, 1.79)]$$

$$\text{Rate of disease among exposed} = \frac{40}{700} = 0.057$$

$$\text{Rate of disease among unexposed} = \frac{30}{920} = 0.033$$

$$\text{Rate ratio} = \frac{0.057}{0.033} = 1.75 \; [95\% \; \text{CI} \; (1.09, 2.81)]$$

$$\text{Rate difference} = 0.057 - 0.033 = 0.024 \; [95\% \; \text{CI} \; (0.00, 0.05)]$$

$$\text{Odds ratio} = \frac{\dfrac{\frac{40}{70}}{\frac{30}{70}}}{\dfrac{\frac{90}{210}}{\frac{120}{210}}} = \frac{40*120}{130*30} = 1.23 \; [95\% \; \text{CI} \; (0.72, 2.10)]$$

FIGURE 9.6 Continued

was estimated given the loss to follow-up and the general ways in which the rate ratio is affected by loss to follow-up.

Non-Comparability When Sampling Is Based on Health Indicator Status

As we detailed in Chapter 4, one way in which to generate a purposive sample is to collect individuals with a health indicator of interest and sample individuals free of the health indicator from the same underlying population base of individuals (a case control study). This is a commonly used design when the disease of interest is rare or the latency period between exposure and disease is long, and thus directly following a group of initially health indicator-free individuals over time to see how many cases arise would require prohibitively large sample sizes and/or long follow-ups.

A case control study can be an efficient way to estimate a measure of the association between exposure and outcome provided that some care is given to the characteristics of the sample. The central considerations of comparability when sampling based on disease status are no different than any other study design: The critical element remains that the exposed and the unexposed are comparable on all other causes of disease. We note for emphasis that even when sampling based on health indicator status, we care about comparability between the exposed and unexposed (not between those with and without the health indicator).

The introduction of non-comparability between exposed and unexposed in a case control study through selection of participants is a common threat to the validity of the design, most often through inappropriate selection of the proper control group for the cases. The non-case group should be selected with the goal that it represents the prevalence of exposure among all non-cases in the underlying population base from which the cases were identified. We cannot empirically validate that the control group we have selected is appropriate, and the consequences of an inappropriate control group are that we estimate the wrong association between exposures and health indicators.

As an example, suppose that we are interested in the potential association between use of dental floss and incidence of gum disease. In the underlying population of Farrlandia in Figure 9.7, we show the incidence of gum disease over 2 years (i.e., among those with no gum disease, we follow individuals for four time points over 2 years and observe who develops gum disease), comparing regular dental floss users (black) with those who do not regularly floss (grey).

In the population, those who regularly use dental floss have 0.25 times the risk, 0.21 times the rate, 0.17 times the odds of developing gum disease over 2 years. Further, regular use of dental floss is associated with 30 fewer cases of gum disease for every 100 people who regularly use it compared with those who do not, and an excess of 8 cases per 100 exposed person years compared with unexposed person years. Note that we do not need confidence intervals when we estimate these associations because we are examining the population rather than a sample of the population.

Of course, we do not have access to the population of Farrlandia. Therefore, we design a study selecting cases with gum disease from several dental clinics in Farrlandia, as well as a proportion of individuals without gum disease from the general population in the same catchment area as the dental clinics. We conceptualize this sample as being selected among the population as it exists at Time 4 in Figure 9.7, that is, with 100 cases eligible to be sampled, and 300 non-cases eligible to be sampled. From those eligible, we select half of the cases and a third of the non-cases thus obtaining a sample of 50 cases and 100 non-cases (Figure 9.8).

Remember from Chapter 7 that because we fixed the marginal totals of diseased and non-diseased in the study sample by sampling a fixed number

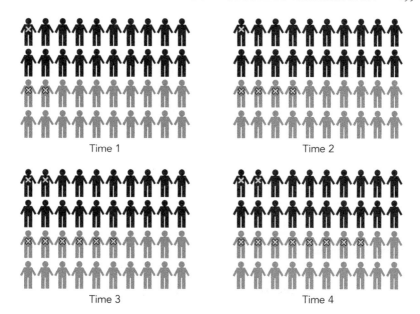

Time 1   Time 2

Time 3   Time 4

2x2 table of association at Time 4

	Health indicator present	Health indicator absent	Total N	Person years
Exposed	20	180	200	950
Unexposed	80	120	200	800
Total N	100	300	400	1750

$$P(D|E+) = \frac{20}{200} = 0.10$$

$$P(D|E-) = \frac{80}{200} = 0.40$$

$$\text{Risk ratio} = \frac{0.10}{0.40} = 0.25$$

$$\text{Risk difference} = 0.10 - 0.40 = -0.3$$

$$\text{Rate of disease among exposed} = \frac{20}{950} = 0.02$$

FIGURE 9.7 Association between dental floss use and gum disease in the population of Farrlandia.

$$\text{Rate of disease among unexposed} = \frac{80}{800} = 0.10$$

$$\text{Rate ratio} = \frac{0.02}{0.10} = 0.21$$

$$\text{Rate difference} = 0.02 - 0.10 = -0.08$$

$$\text{Odds ratio} = \frac{\dfrac{\dfrac{20}{100}}{\dfrac{80}{100}}}{\dfrac{\dfrac{180}{300}}{\dfrac{120}{300}}} = \frac{20*120}{180*80} = 0.17$$

FIGURE 9.7 Continued

of cases and non-cases, the risk of disease no longer has interpretive meaning. Thus, we use the odds ratio as the measure of association:

$$\text{Odds ratio} = \frac{\dfrac{\dfrac{10}{50}}{\dfrac{40}{50}}}{\dfrac{\dfrac{60}{100}}{\dfrac{40}{100}}} = \frac{10*40}{60*40} = 0.17, \ 95\% \text{ CI } [0.07, 0.37]$$

We obtain the same point estimate for the odds ratio in the study sample that we would have obtained with access to the underlying population base in

	Health indicator present	Health indicator absent	Total N
Exposed	10	60	70
Unexposed	40	40	80
Total N	50	100	150

FIGURE 9.8 Sample selection for study of dental floss use and gum disease.

Farrlandia. This is because we sampled the cases and non-cases from an underlying prospectively followed group and selected the same proportion of exposed and unexposed within those who have the disease and those who do not.

This illustrates a central principle in the conduct of studies in which the sampling strategy is to select cases and non-cases: We must conceptualize an underlying population of people that produced the cases and non-cases. As long as we sample the cases and non-cases from this underlying dynamic group in such a way that the sampling is the same in exposure groups (e.g., in our example we selected 50% of exposed and unexposed individuals with the disease and 30% of exposed and unexposed individuals without the disease), then we obtain an unbiased estimate of the odds ratio.

What can go wrong when we are selecting based on disease status? We get a biased estimate of the odds ratio if we sample differently based on exposure status. For example, imagine that we selected our non-cases not from the underlying population of Farrlandia but from individuals at the dental clinics who did not have gum disease. Individuals who regularly go to the dentist may be more likely to use dental floss than individuals who do not regularly go to the dentist. Thus, we may get a higher proportion of dental floss users in the sample of people without gum disease than we would see in the underlying population of Farrlandia. This would constitute sampling differently by exposure status in the case and non-case group, rendering a biased estimate of the odds ratio. In the scenario in which controls were selected from the dental clinic, we would expect the association between dental floss use and gum disease to be underestimated because we overestimate the probability of exposure among the controls.

Because control selection in case control studies can so often go wrong, we consider another example to fully illustrate the fundamentals. We are interested in the association between a genetic risk factor and the development of prostate cancer over 20 years among men age 60 to 80. The true association in the underlying population of Farrlandia is shown in Figure 9.9.

In the underlying population of Farrlandia, men with the genetic factor have 2.5 times the risk, 2.64 times the rate, and 2.8 times the odds of prostate cancer over 10 years compared with those who lack the genetic factor. Having the genetic factor is associated with an additional 10 cases of prostate cancer per 100 men exposed compared with unexposed, and an excess rate of prostate cancer of about 5.7 cases per 1,000 person years associated with the exposure.

As always, however, we do not have access to the population; we need to take a sample. We select newly diagnosed prostate cancer cases from the five hospitals in the Farrlandia. For the comparison group, we select other cancer patients at the hospital who do not have prostate cancer. Unbeknownst

	Health indicator present	Health indicator absent	Total N	Person years
Exposed	500	2500	3000	54750
Unexposed	200	2800	3000	57900
Total N	700	5300	6000	112650

$$P(D|E+) = \frac{500}{3000} = 0.17$$

$$P(D|E-) = \frac{200}{2800} = 0.17$$

$$\text{Risk ratio} = \frac{0.17}{0.07} = 2.50$$

$$\text{Risk difference} = 0.17 - 0.07 = 0.10$$

$$\text{Rate of disease among exposed} = \frac{500}{54750} = 0.00913$$

$$\text{Rate of disease among unexposed} = \frac{200}{57900} = 0.00345$$

$$\text{Rate ratio} = \frac{0.00913}{0.00345} = 2.64$$

$$\text{Rate difference} = 0.00913 - 0.00345 = 0.00568$$

$$\text{Odds ratio} = \frac{\dfrac{\frac{500}{700}}{\frac{200}{700}}}{\dfrac{\frac{2500}{5300}}{\frac{2800}{5300}}} = \frac{500 * 2800}{2500 * 200} = 2.80$$

FIGURE 9.9 Association between the genetic risk factor and prostate cancer in the population.

to us, however, this genetic factor is associated with multiple cancer sites in addition to the prostate. Thus, cancer cases are more likely to have this genetic factor compared with the underlying population of individuals without prostate cancer in Farrlandia. The study data we obtain are shown in Figure 9.10.

	Health indicator present	Health indicator absent	Total N
Exposed	50	500	550
Unexposed	20	280	300
Total N	70	780	850

$$\text{Odds ratio} = \frac{\dfrac{\dfrac{50}{70}}{\dfrac{20}{70}}}{\dfrac{\dfrac{500}{780}}{\dfrac{280}{780}}} = \frac{50*280}{500*20} = 1.40 \; [95\% \; CI \; (0.82, 2.40)]$$

FIGURE 9.10 Association between the genetic factor and prostate cancer in a sample.

In our study sample, men with the genetic factor have 1.4 times the odds of prostate cancer compared with men with other cancers who do not have the genetic factor. Compared with the truth in Farrlandia, we see that we have underestimated the true odds of prostate cancer in the underlying Farrlandia population.

Why did this happen? Note that in the underlying population of interest, among those without prostate cancer, 47% had the genetic factor (2,500/5,300). In our study sample, 64% had the genetic factor. Thus, there is a greater proportion of exposed individuals among non-cases (note that non-cases in this study indicates no prostate cancer) compared with the non-diseased in the underlying population of interest. Because of this overrepresentation of the genetic factor among the non-cases in the study sample, we underestimate the true association between the genetic factor and prostate cancer.

This bias occurred because of non-comparability between exposed and unexposed (not case and non-case). In this example, those unexposed no longer represent the disease experience of the exposed if they had not been exposed.

To summarize comparability when sampling based on disease status, for a non-biased estimate of the odds ratio in the underlying population of interest, the non-cases in the sample should have the same probability of exposure as non-cases in the underlying base of individuals from which the cases were drawn. Note that without some type of nested case control design (see online material that accompanies this chapter for more detail on nested designs) we can never confirm whether the non-cases in our sample indeed have the same probability of exposure as non-cases in the underlying population from which the cases were drawn; thus, it is critical to conceptualize a study base from which cases and non-cases are drawn and select these case and non-case groups to represent the exposure probabilities of each group from within this underlying base.

Source of Non-Comparability: Misclassification

Careful and accurate measurement of potential exposures, outcomes, confounders, and other variables of interest are critical to the success of an epidemiologic study. Even the most perfectly designed study with excellent participation and follow-up rates can be undone by poor measurement of key variables of interest. Specifically, measurement error can lead to non-comparability in our observed exposure–outcome relationship, which as we have learned can cause improper inference about the exposure–disease relationship. In this section, we describe how errors in measurement can affect our measures of exposure–outcome relations, and we describe some fundamental principles for improving measurement accuracy.

We use as an example a hypothetical study of the association between coffee consumption and risk of stroke among women. Available evidence indicates that coffee consumption is associated with reduced risk of stroke among women in the United States (Larsson, Virtamo, & Wolk, 2011; Lopez-Garcia et al., 2009). In data drawn from a prospective study of incident strokes, women who consumed more than four cups of coffee per day had 0.80 times the risk of an incident stroke; remember, when examining relative associations, 1.0 is indicative of no association, and anything less than 1.0 indicates that those exposed are less likely to develop the health indicator. Our risk ratio of 0.80 is less than 1.0, indicating that those who drink >4 cups of coffee have a lower risk than those who drink less than or equal to 4 cups. Overall, the data suggest that coffee consumption is potentially protective for the development of this outcome.

Suppose that we conduct a study of coffee drinking and stroke among women in Farrlandia. Following are the data from the population without any measurement error of any kind. For the example, the population of interest consists of 4,000 women age 60 and older with no history of stroke, observed over 1 year. Again, because we are using the whole population, there is no loss to follow-up and no confidence intervals are necessary. Note that we never actually know the true population data, only what we are able to measure; thus, these data are entirely hypothetical. For simplicity, in Figure 9.11 we

	Health indicator present	Health indicator absent	Total N	Person years
Exposed	500	1500	2000	1750
Unexposed	1000	1000	2000	1500
Total N	1500	2500	4000	3250

$$P(D|E+) = \frac{500}{2000} = 0.25$$

$$P(D|E-) = \frac{1000}{2000} = 0.50$$

$$\text{Risk ratio} = \frac{0.25}{0.5} = 0.50$$

$$\text{Risk difference} = 0.25 - 0.50 = -0.25$$

$$\text{Rate of disease among exposed} = \frac{500}{1750} = 0.29$$

$$\text{Rate of disease among unexposed} = \frac{1000}{1500} = 0.67$$

$$\text{Rate ratio} = \frac{0.29}{0.67} = 0.43$$

$$\text{Rate difference} = 0.29 - 0.67 = -0.38$$

$$\text{Odds ratio} = \frac{\dfrac{\dfrac{500}{1500}}{\dfrac{1000}{1500}}}{\dfrac{\dfrac{1500}{2500}}{\dfrac{1000}{2500}}} = \frac{500 * 1000}{1500 * 1000} = 0.33$$

FIGURE 9.11 Association between coffee consumption and risk of stroke in the population of Farrlandia.

compare heavy coffee drinkers (>4 cups/day, on average) to all others in the population (less than or equal to 4 cups/day, on average).

Thus, individuals drinking >4 cups/day have 0.5 times the risk and 0.43 times the rate of stroke compared with women who do not consume >4 cups/day over 1 year. We would expect 25 fewer cases of stroke for every 100 coffee drinkers, or 6.7 fewer cases for every 100 person years of exposure that is associated with coffee drinking. Finally, the odds of stroke over 1 year for heavy coffee users are 0.33 times that of non-heavy users. Note that the odds ratio is not a good approximation of the risk ratio in this case because stroke in this population is common (1,500/4,000 = 0.375 or 37.5%).

Our Sample

From the population of Farrlandia, we take a representative sample of 400 women with no history of stroke. We ask the women how much coffee they consume on average every day. We then follow the women forward for 1 year, counting how many cases of stroke arise among the heavy coffee drinkers and the non-heavy drinkers. At the end of 1 year, we compare the incidence of stroke between the two groups. But our measure of coffee consumption is based on the report of the women themselves, and it is likely that some women misreported their coffee consumption. How will this affect our results?

A Basic Understanding of Measurement Error

We now use these data to describe how various types of measurement errors can affect our estimates of association. Measurement error broadly refers to mistakes in how we record an individual's value on a variable of interest in our study. These mistakes can arise from numerous sources. Respondents may not report accurately, a diagnostic test used may have errors in it, or there may be problems in coding the responses into a database. All of these sources lead to measurement error. Errors can take several different forms: (a) error can be random; (b) error can be associated with exposure status but not outcome status; or alternatively, (c) with outcome status but not exposure status; or (d) error can be associated with both outcome and exposure status. Random measurement error will generally lead to imprecision and underestimation of associations, and we do not go into detail about it in this chapter.

In Figure 9.12, we describe how we notate measurement error in this chapter. We notate error with reference to the "truth"—remember, we happen to know the truth in Farrlandia; but in reality, we never know

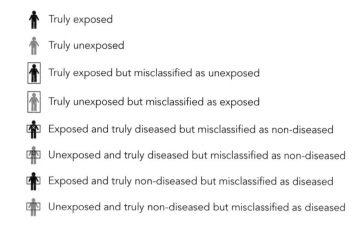

FIGURE 9.12 Misclassification notation.

the true exposure status of our study participants, only their measured exposure status.

Errors That Are Associated With Exposure Status or Disease Status, but Not Both

Measurement error can be random but is often not random. A classic example of this is the scale that is 5 pounds off. Suppose we are conducting a study of whether body weight predicts diabetes onset, and we use an old scale that is not properly calibrated. Every individual in the study is measured as being 5 pounds more than they actually weigh. This would lead to misclassification of the exposure: weight. It is not random, because every individual is recorded as 5 pounds heavier than they actually weigh (rather than an approximately equal proportion of individuals recorded as 5 pounds heavier vs. 5 pounds lighter). Rather, this error is systematic and associated with exposure status.

How does misclassification associated with exposure status affect our estimates? We return to our example of coffee consumption and stroke. Shown in Figure 9.13 is our sample from Farrlandia with misclassification related to exposure status. Each individual in Figure 9.13 represents the experience of 10 individuals (thus, the 40 individuals shown in Figure 9.13 represent 400 individuals). Suppose that half of the women who were truly exposed (drank >4 cups/day, on average) reported that they were unexposed (drank less than or equal to 4 cups/day, on average). No women who were truly ≤4 cup-a-day drinkers reported drinking more than 4 cups. We would obtain the data shown in Figures 9.13.

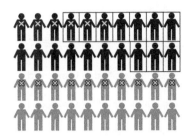

	Health indicator present	Health indicator absent	Total N	Person years
Exposed	30	70	100	85
Unexposed	100 + 30 = 130	100 + 70 = 170	300	235
Total N	160	240	400	320

$$P(D|E+) = \frac{30}{100} = 0.3$$

$$P(D|E-) = \frac{130}{300} = 0.43$$

$$\text{Risk ratio} = \frac{0.3}{0.43} = 0.69 \ [95\% \ CI \ (0.50, 0.96)]$$

$$\text{Risk difference} = 0.3 - 0.43 = 0.13 \ [95\% \ CI \ (-.24, -0.03)]$$

$$\text{Rate of disease among exposed} = \frac{30}{85} = 0.35$$

$$\text{Rate of disease among unexposed} = \frac{130}{235} = 0.55$$

$$\text{Rate ratio} = \frac{0.35}{0.55} = 0.64 \ [95\% \ CI \ (0.43, 0.95)]$$

$$\text{Rate difference} = 0.35 - 0.55 = -0.20 [95\% \ CI \ (-0.36, -0.04)]$$

$$\text{Odds ratio} = \frac{\dfrac{\frac{30}{160}}{\frac{130}{160}}}{\dfrac{\frac{70}{240}}{\frac{170}{240}}} = \frac{30*170}{70*130} = 0.56 [95\% \ CI \ (0.35, 0.91)]$$

FIGURE 9.13 The association between coffee consumption and stroke when there is misclassification of coffee consumption status.

We would report that heavy coffee drinking in women over age 60 is associated with 0.69 times the risk of stroke over 1 year. Further, approximately 13 cases of stroke per 100 women would be prevented if all women drank more than 4 cups per day. Finally, the odds of stroke over 1 year among heavy coffee drinking women is 0.56 times that of light/no coffee drinking.

Thus, the effect of misclassification of exposure status is that we underestimate the magnitude of the protective relation between coffee drinking and stroke. That is, the observed association is closer to a null association (risk, rate, and odds ratio of 1.0, risk and rate difference of 0). We provide a quantitative example of misclassification of health indicator status that is independent of exposure status in Box 9.5 of the online material that accompanies this chapter. Together, these examples illustrate a fundamental principle of misclassification that is related to exposure status but not to health indicator status, or related to health indicator status but not to exposure status: In most cases, this type of misclassification will render results that are underestimates of the true association, whether more exposed are misclassified as unexposed, or vice versa, and whether those with the health indicators are misclassified as not having the health indicator, or vice versa. The broader principle is, again, that the misclassification leads to non-comparability between the exposed and the unexposed.

Errors That Are Associated With Both Exposure Status and Disease Status

Misclassification of exposure status can be linked to health indicator status, and similarly, misclassification of health indicator status can be linked to exposure status. To understand how this type of misclassification results in non-comparability, we work through an example.

In Farrlandia, we are interested in whether there is a causal effect of using over-the-counter cold medication in pregnancy with congenital malformations in neonates. The population of interest is all neonates born over a 3-year period. If we were able to observe the truth in the population, which for our purposes consists of 3,000 Farrlandians, we would observe the data found in Figure 9.14.

In truth, there is no association between cold medicine use and congenital malformations. We see in the population that 33.3% of women used cold medicine during pregnancy, and an equal proportion of neonates developed congenital malformations in the exposed and unexposed groups. We did not

	Health indicator present	Health indicator absent	Total N
Exposed	10	990	1000
Unexposed	20	1980	2000
Total N	30	2970	3000

$$P(D|E+) = \frac{10}{1000} = 0.01$$

$$P(D|E-) = \frac{20}{2000} = 0.01$$

$$\text{Risk ratio} = \frac{0.01}{0.01} = 1.00$$

$$\text{Risk difference} = 0.01 - 0.01 = 0.00$$

$$\text{Odds ratio} = \frac{\dfrac{\dfrac{10}{30}}{\dfrac{20}{30}}}{\dfrac{\dfrac{990}{2970}}{\dfrac{1980}{2970}}} = \frac{10*1980}{990*20} = 1.00[95\% \text{ CI } (0.47,2.14)]$$

FIGURE 9.14 Association between cold medicine and congenital malformations in the population.

estimate rates, rate ratios, or rate differences for this example because the period between pregnancy and birth is relatively short.

We do not have access to the whole population of Farrlandia, however, so we need to take a sample. Our sampling strategy is to take all cases of neo-nates with congenital malformations in the five hospitals in Farrlandia across the 3 years. We ascertain all 30 cases in the population. We also sample 300 healthy newborns from the same hospitals at the same time frame. We ask the mothers whether they used any cold medication in pregnancy.

In our study sample, if we were able to measure cold medicine use perfectly, we would observe the data found in Figure 9.15.

Remember from Chapter 6 that because we fixed the marginal totals of diseased and non-diseased in the study sample by sampling a fixed number of

	Health indicator present	Health indicator absent	Total N
Exposed	10	100	110
Unexposed	20	200	220
Total N	30	300	330

FIGURE 9.15 Association between cold medicine and congenital malformations in the sample.

cases and non-cases, the risk of disease no longer has interpretive causal meaning. Thus, we use the ratio of odds as the measure of association.

$$\text{Odds ratio} = \frac{\dfrac{\dfrac{10}{110}}{\dfrac{100}{110}}}{\dfrac{\dfrac{20}{220}}{\dfrac{200}{220}}} = \frac{10*200}{100*20} = 1.00,\ 95\%\ \text{CI}\ [0.45, 2.22]$$

The odds of congenital malformations in offspring of women who used cold medicine is equal to the odds of congenital malformations in the offspring of women who did not. The sample data with perfect measurement are reflective of the population association, as shown in Figure 9.14.

What if, however, we introduce misclassification of the exposure status? Women who have children with congenital malformations may search their memories for potential reasons that their infants were afflicted. Women who have healthy newborns, on the other hand, may not remember their pregnancy exposures as well and may be more likely to report not using cold medicine when in fact they did. In the scenario in Figure 9.16, we have misclassified the exposure status; and further, mothers of cases are more likely to accurately report their exposure status compared with mothers of non-cases. How would this affect our estimates?

FIGURE 9.16 Association between cold medicine and congenital malformations—misclassification of exposure status dependent on disease status.

If half of the exposed women from the non-case group report no exposure when in fact they were exposed, we would observe that use of cold medicine in pregnancy is associated with a 2.5 times increase in the odds of congenital malformations when in fact there is no relationship. In this scenario, we are underestimating the exposure probability in the non-case group compared with the truth in the study sample, leading to an overestimation of the effect of the exposure on the outcome.

We could posit a different misclassification scenario, however. Suppose that women in the case group underreported their cold medicine use for fear of being blamed for the child's condition. Women in the non-case group, in contrast, reported their cold medicine use accurately. The data are presented in Figure 9.17.

In this scenario, half of the women in the case group who used cold medicine reported that they did not use cold medicine, whereas women in the non-case group reported accurately. Under this scenario, it appears that cold medicine is potentially protective against the development of congenital malformations, as women who reported using cold medicine

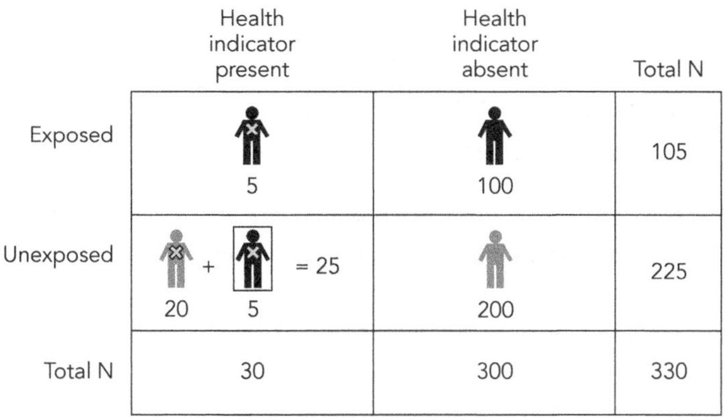

	Health indicator present	Health indicator absent	Total N
Exposed	5	100	105
Unexposed	20 + 5 = 25	200	225
Total N	30	300	330

$$\text{Odds ratio} = \frac{\dfrac{\frac{5}{30}}{\frac{25}{30}}}{\dfrac{\frac{100}{300}}{\frac{200}{300}}} = \frac{5*200}{100*25} = 0.40 \; [95\% \; CI \; (0.15, 1.08)]$$

FIGURE 9.17 Association between cold medicine and congenital malformations—misclassification of exposure dependent on health indicator status.

had 0.4 times the odds of having a child with a malformation compared to women who did not. In this scenario, we are underestimating the exposure probability in the case group compared with the truth in the study sample, leading to an underestimation of the effect of the exposure on the outcome.

In summary, errors in classification that are associated with both exposure and disease status can create non-comparability in the observed data, leading to incorrect inference. The direction of the bias will depend on which groups are more likely to be misclassified.

We note that the examples in this section were regarding misclassification of exposure status, but misclassification of disease status dependent on exposure can and does occur (see Box 9.5 of the online material that accompanies Chapter 9). Similar to situations in which exposure is misclassified dependent on disease status, the resulting bias could render either overestimation or underestimation of the measure of association.

In Box 9.1, we provide an overview of some of the common ways in which misclassification arises in epidemiologic studies.

BOX 9.1

Some Common Ways in Which Misclassification Arises, in No Particular Order

No matter how the misclassification arises, it will result in biased estimates of the association between exposure and disease to the extent that non-comparability between the exposed and unexposed arises as a result of the misclassification process. Following are three common ways in which misclassification arises.

- We conduct a study of the effects of using a particular medication on a secondary unintended outcome. We may detect more cases of the outcome in the medication group because they see physicians more regularly (e.g., to obtain prescription refills); thus, there are more opportunities for diagnosis of secondary health outcomes.
- We conduct a study where we sample individuals with a particular disease and compare them to individuals without that disease. Study investigators directly conduct the interviews with patients. We spend more time with the diseased individuals and ask more questions about potential exposures because we are sure that our hypothesis is correct.
- Individuals with a particular disease of interest may be better reporters of their past exposures, as they are more invested in finding out the cause of their disease.

Summary

Non-comparability in epidemiologic studies arises when the exposed and unexposed groups do not have an even distribution of other causes of the health indicator of interest. There are four main ways that non-comparability can arise: 1) by chance; 2) because causes are associated with one another; 3) when selecting or following eligible study participants; or 4) through mis-classification of study variables. Sometimes we can predict whether these types of bias will render observed estimates that are larger or smaller than what we would expect the true population association to be, but some-times we cannot predict the direction of the bias. Careful study design, and rigorous and comprehensive measurement are the keys to reducing non-comparability. We note, however, that almost all studies will suffer from at least some non-comparability—the critical job for the epidemiologist is to decide how much non-comparability is evident in the sample, the source of the non-comparability, and to execute strategies to reduce the effects of non-comparability. In the next chapter, we address this last point, guiding the student through common strategies for reducing non-comparability.

Note

1. We note that some evidence indicates that cigarette smoking and alcohol consumption interact to cause esophageal cancer in some individuals (Castellsague et al., 1999). That is, as introduced in Chapter 7, alcohol and tobacco may be component causes in the same set that produces disease. In Chapter 11, we provide a comprehensive overview of interaction in epidemiologic studies. For simplicity in this example, we proceed without considering the potential interaction of alcohol consumption and cigarette smoking.

References

Blot, W. J. (1992). Alcohol and cancer. *Cancer Research, 52*(Suppl. 7), 2119s–2123s.

Castellsague, X., Munoz, N., De Stefani, E., Victora, C. G., Castelletto, R., Rolon, P. A., & Quintana, M. J. (1999). Independent and joint effects of tobacco smoking and alcohol drinking on the risk of esophageal cancer in men and women. *International Journal of Cancer, 82*, 657–664.

Choi, S. Y., & Kahyo, H. (1991). Effect of cigarette smoking and alcohol consumption in the etiology of cancers of the digestive tract. *International Journal of Cancer, 49*, 381–386.

Connor, J. (2006). The life and times of the J-shaped curve. *Alcohol and Alcoholism, 41*, 583–584.

Franceschi, S., Talamini, R., Barra, S., Baron, A. E., Negri, E., Bidoli, E., . . . La Vecchia, C. (1990). Smoking and drinking in relation to cancers of the oral cavity, pharynx, larynx, and esophagus in northern Italy. *Cancer Research, 50*, 6502–6507.

Hasin, D. S., Stinson, F. S., Ogburn, E., & Grant, B. F. (2007). Prevalence, correlates, disability, and comorbidity of DSM-IV alcohol abuse and dependence in the United States: Results from the National Epidemiologic Survey on Alcohol and Related Conditions. *Archives of General Psychiatry, 64*, 830–842.

Larsson, S. C., Virtamo, J., & Wolk, A. (2011). Coffee consumption and risk of stroke in women. *Stroke, 42*, 908–912.

Lopez-Garcia, E., Rodriguez-Artalejo, F., Rexrode, K. M., Logroscino, G., Hu, F. B., & van Dam, R. M. (2009). Coffee consumption and risk of stroke in women. *Circulation, 119*, 1116–1123.

10

How Can We Mitigate Against Noncausal Associations in Design and Analysis?

WE CONTINUE IN this chapter to explore Step 5 in our seven-step process of the foundations of epidemiologic studies. Having explicated how we think of causes in epidemiology, how comparability between exposed and unexposed is an important component of our ability to make strong conclusions from our data, and the central ways in which non-comparability arises when we conduct epidemiologic studies, we now conclude our assessment of Step 5 by describing three foundational ways in which comparability is achieved in epidemiologic studies: (a) randomize individuals to receive the exposure or not, (b) match individuals in the study to each other on variables that are potential causes of non-comparability, and (c) stratify the data to determine whether there is an association between exposure and outcome holding constant variables contributing to non-comparability. We note that these approaches to mitigating the effects of non-comparability are not comprehensive of all approaches and that these approaches do not apply to all sources of non-comparability (e.g., those resulting from loss to follow-up that are related to health indicators of interest, or to misclassification); nevertheless, they are foundational epidemiologic methods for mastery at an introductory level.

Randomization

Randomization is a powerful way to create comparability between groups. A major source of non-comparability in epidemiologic studies is that those who choose to, for example, smoke, also are likely to engage in other behaviors with adverse consequences for health. When we randomize, we remove the individual's ability to choose an exposure status. This study design is known as the *randomized controlled trial* (RCT), and the samples are almost always purposive. That is, individuals are selected into the study based on eligibility criteria and then randomized to receive the exposure or not. We then follow them forward to determine who develops the health indicators of interest and who does not. RCT study samples are generally not randomly selected to achieve representativeness of an underlying population. Further, RCTs are always longitudinal cohort studies in which individuals are followed forward in time, with outcomes assessed at multiple time points during the course of the study.

Why is randomization a way to control for non-comparability? Suppose two investigators conduct two separate studies on the effects of vitamin A consumption on the incidence of cardiovascular disease among post-menopausal women, hypothesizing that the vitamin is protective against cardiovascular disease. The first investigator collects a purposive sample of 80 postmenopausal women with no history of cardiovascular disease. She asks the women whether they regularly take a vitamin A supplement. She follows them by exposure status (whether they take the vitamin or not) and then follows them forward for 5 years, counting the number in each group who have a cardiovascular event. Assume no loss to follow-up. Figure 10.1 contains the 2 × 2 table of her results.

The risk of cardiovascular disease among those who took the vitamin is 20%. The risk of cardiovascular disease among those who did not take the vitamin is much higher, 40%. Based on these results, postmenopausal women who take vitamin A have approximately 0.5 times the risk (that is, about half of the risk) and 0.38 times the odds of cardiovascular disease compared with those who do not take vitamin A, and there are approximately 20 fewer cases of cardiovascular disease per every 100 women who take vitamin A compared with those who do not over 5 years. Are we concerned about the validity of her results? Well, those who choose to take vitamin supplements may be less likely to smoke, may eat a more healthful diet, exercise, and so forth. Without taking these factors into consideration, we do not know whether the vitamin A had any causal effect on their cardiovascular health at all. In fact, when the investigator looked in her data at the measures of diet, she found that the vitamin takers had much lower average daily saturated fat intake than the non-takers. Figure 10.2 is her study sample, with the dots now reflecting those who have more saturated fat in their daily diet than recommended levels.

	Health indicator present	Health indicator absent	Total N
Exposed	8	32	40
Unexposed	16	24	40
Total N	24	56	80

$$P(D|E+) = \frac{8}{40} = 0.20$$

$$P(D|E-) = \frac{16}{40} = 0.40$$

$$\text{Risk ratio} = \frac{0.20}{0.40} = 0.50 \ [95\% \ CI(0.24, 1.03)]$$

$$\text{Risk difference} = 0.2 - 0.4 = -0.20 \ [95\% \ CI(-0.40, 0.00)]$$

$$\text{Odds ratio} = \frac{\dfrac{\frac{8}{24}}{\frac{16}{24}}}{\dfrac{\frac{32}{56}}{\frac{24}{56}}} = \frac{8*24}{32*16} = 0.38 \ [95\% \ CI \ (0.14, 1.02)]$$

FIGURE 10.1 Observational study of the association between vitamin A use and cardiovascular disease.

When we count the number of people with dots among the vitamin takers and non-takers, we see that there are 9 dotted people (high fat consumers) among the 40 vitamin takers, for a total prevalence of 22.5% of high fat consumption among the vitamin takers. In contrast, among the 40 non-takers, the prevalence of high saturated fat diet is 45%. Thus, there is a greater proportion of high fat consumers among the non-takers. This is just one of myriad differences that make vitamin takers different than non-takers. It would be exceedingly difficult to measure all of the factors that may differ between these groups and to take account of them in a rigorous way. Yet the question of whether vitamin A use is heart healthy is one of potentially great public health importance. What can be done?

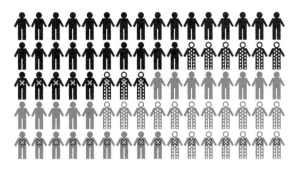

FIGURE 10.2 Sample of 80 postmenopausal women regarding vitamin A use (black), saturated fat intake (dots), and cardiovascular disease (X): observational study.

The second investigator also collects a purposive sample of 80 women with no history of heart disease but randomly assigns them to take either vitamin A or a placebo pill that looked and tasted just like vitamin A. Similarly to the first investigator, she follows the women over 5 years and counts the number of cardiovascular events and has no loss to follow-up. Figure 10.3 contains is the 2 × 2 table of her results.

We see that the risk of cardiovascular disease among those randomized to take vitamin A is almost the same as the risk of cardiovascular disease among those in the placebo group over 5 years (a risk ratio of 0.98, odds ratio of 0.97, and risk difference of −0.01). Do we have the same concern about the effects of poor diet, smoking, and other factors in the randomized study that we did in the observational study? Surely some of the individuals in the study smoke, eat diets rich in saturated fat, and so forth. How do these factors play out in the randomized trial? We evaluate it empirically. Similar to the first study, the second investigator also measured the proportion of individuals with an average daily intake of saturated fat above recommended levels. In Figure 10.4, we present the data from the randomized trial, using dots to indicate high fat consumption.

Now, when we count the number of people with dots among the vitamin A takers and non-takers, we see that there are 12 dotted people (high fat consumers) among the 40 vitamin A takers, for a total prevalence of 30%. Among the 40 non-takers, the total prevalence is also 30%. Thus, the same proportion of vitamin A takers and non-takers consume a high fat diet. Given that the high fat diet is evenly distributed across groups, it will not affect the internal validity of the study estimate.

This is the advantage of randomization. All factors that would differ between two groups who were able to choose their exposure status are, on

	Health indicator present	Health indicator absent	Total N
Exposed	12	24	36
Unexposed	15	29	44
Total N	27	53	80

$$P(D|E+) = \frac{12}{36} = 0.33$$

$$P(D|E-) = \frac{15}{44} = 0.34$$

$$\text{Risk ratio} = \frac{0.33}{0.34} = 0.98 \; [95\% \; CI \; (0.53, 1.81)]$$

$$\text{Risk difference} = 0.33 - 0.34 = -0.01 \; [95\% \; CI \; (-0.22, 0.20)]$$

$$\text{Odds ratio} = \frac{\dfrac{\frac{12}{27}}{\frac{15}{27}}}{\dfrac{\frac{24}{53}}{\frac{29}{53}}} = \frac{12*29}{24*15} = 0.97 \; [95\% \; CI \; (0.38, 2.46)]$$

FIGURE 10.3 Randomized study of the association between vitamin A use and cardiovascular disease.

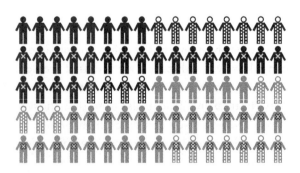

FIGURE 10.4 Sample of 80 postmenopausal women regarding vitamin A use (black), saturated fat intake (dots), and cardiovascular disease (X): randomized study.

average, evenly distributed between the groups when randomly assigned to exposure status. This includes all factors that are known to be associated with the health indicator of interest (thus, for cardiovascular disease, we might be concerned about diet, smoking, exercise, other medication, and substance use) and the myriad of unknown or difficult to measure factors that differ between vitamin takers and non-takers. Even when we cannot ethically randomize an exposure, we search for opportunities in which exposures were largely outside of the control of individuals to approximate the conditions of a randomized trial. In Box 10.1 of the online material that accompanies this chapter, we provide an overview and examples of such studies, termed natural experiments.

Compliance and Intention to Treat Analysis, Loss to Follow-Up

Special issues arise when analyzing data from randomized trials. Even if we can ethically randomize participants to a certain exposure, we often have few guarantees that the individuals in the study will comply with the randomization. In our vitamin study, for example, some people randomized to take the vitamin may not comply with their random assignment and may stop taking it. Some individuals in the non-vitamin group may go on a health kick and pick up some multivitamins at the store. Further, some individuals will inevitably drop out of our study, for reasons that may or may not be related to their treatment assignment, their eventual outcome, or both.

In many randomized trials, there will be participants who do not comply with treatment protocol and/or switch treatment protocols. Remember the Women's Health Initiative study detailed in Box 8.1 of Chapter 8, a large randomized trial assessing the effects of hormone replacement therapy on outcomes such as stroke and cancer. In the course of the study, 42% of women randomly assigned to receive hormone replacement and 38% of the women assigned to placebo stopped taking their regimens during the study follow-up (Rossouw et al., 2002). Further, some women initiated hormone use through their personal clinicians.

Yet the main findings of the study are based on the original groups that these women were randomized into, even if some of the women spent more time not taking the assigned protocol than taking the assigned protocol. Why? The advantage of randomization as a means to control non-comparability is based on the principle that the randomization itself creates comparability between the groups. The women who stop taking their assigned protocols or start taking non-assigned protocols are likely different in ways that affect their risk of the outcomes. In short, if we compared women based on whether they took their assigned treatment, these women may no longer be comparable. Only the original treatment assignment groups have the potential to be comparable across both known and unknown causes of the health indicator. To preserve the comparability generated by randomization and attain a valid effect estimate, we base our analysis on original group membership. This estimate is called the intention-to-treat estimate because it represents our original intention in the study to either treat the participant with an active treatment or a placebo.

Finally, loss to follow-up is a potential threat to validity in the randomized trial, especially if losses to follow-up are related to both the treatment assignment and the outcome. For example, if women assigned to hormone replacement therapy dropped out of the study due to side effects of the hormone drugs, and these women who dropped out where more likely to have health problems than women who stayed in the study, our estimates of association would be biased. Randomization cannot cure non-comparability that arises in longitudinal studies due to drop out that is differential by exposure and outcome.

In Box 10.2 of the online material that accompanies Chapter 10, we review other limitations and design considerations critical to consider in randomized controlled studies: equipoise and ethics, placebos and placebo effects, and the importance of blinding.

Matching

Randomization is an impressive tool to control non-comparability in epidemiologic studies, but it is often unethical and unfeasible. Thus, we need additional tools to control non-comparability in studies where randomization is not possible.

Matching participants on potential sources of non-comparability is one common way in which to control for non-comparability in the design stage of the study. In studies in which individuals free of the health indicator of interest are sampled based on exposure status and followed forward in time (cohort studies), an exposed individual can be matched to one or more unexposed individuals based on one or more factors of interest. More common, however, is to match individuals with a health indicator of interest to individuals free of the health indicator individuals in a case control design.

As an example, suppose that we conduct a study investigating whether low intake of fish oil in the diet is associated an increase in the risk of depression. We collect a sample of 25 individuals with a first diagnosis of depression from a local mental health treatment center. We also collect 25 individuals with no history of depression from the community surrounding the mental health treatment center.

We may be concerned about sex as a potential source of non-comparability in this association. Women are more likely to develop depression compared with men, and women on average have more nutritious diets and may be more likely to supplement their diets with fish oil. Thus, any association between fish oil consumption and depression will be confounded by sex. We might also be concerned about other potential sources of non-comparability such as age, use of substances such as alcohol and cigarettes, and socioeconomic factors, among other potentially relevant exposures, but we focus for now on sex only.

Typically in such case control studies, we have many more potential controls than cases. Thus, each time we select a case from the treatment center, we determine whether the case is a man or woman and select one or more controls of the same sex. Suppose that Figure 10.5 contains our study data.

We have 27 individuals who are low consumers of fish oil (exposed, black) and 23 individuals who are high consumers of fish oil (unexposed, grey). Each case of depression is matched to a control of the same sex, with men denoted with dots and women denoted with no dots.

Thus, there is an equal distribution of sex among those with depression and those without, by design, because each case was matched to a control of

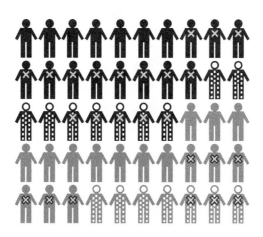

FIGURE 10.5 Using matching to control non-comparability.

the same sex. If two thirds of the individuals in the sample with depression are women, then by design, two thirds of the sample without depression will also be women.

We can now conceptualize this sample not as 50 individuals but 25 pairs. Each pair is identical with respect to the matched factors. In our example, this is sex, so each pair consists of 2 women or 2 men. In Figure 10.6 we show a visualization of the matching process. Once data are matched, we can consider them as pairs or groups (if matching more than one case or more than one control) rather than individuals.

Now that we have matched pairs of data, our traditional 2 × 2 table of exposure and disease changes to a 2 × 2 table of the matched pairs. Each individual in the matched pair is either exposed or unexposed to the relevant exposure of interest. The row of the matched-pair 2 × 2 will be the exposure status of one member of the pair, and the column of the matched-pair 2 × 2 will be the exposure status of the other member of the pair. In Figure 10.7, we have four kinds of matched pairs in each of our four cells: Either the case and the control are both exposed, the case is exposed but the control is not, the control is exposed but the case is not, or both are unexposed.

Consider our study sample examining the association between fish oil consumption and depression, matched on sex in Figure 10.7. In the upper left-hand corner we have six pairs in which both the depressed and non-depressed

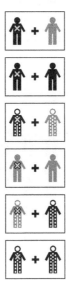

FIGURE 10.6 How to match pairs.

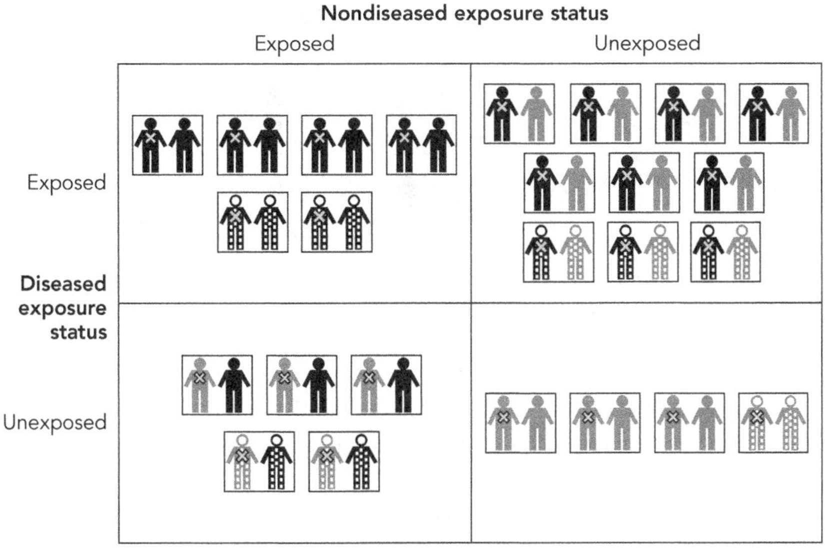

FIGURE 10.7 Association between fish oil consumption and depression, matched on sex.

individuals were low consumers of fish oil. Four of these pairs were women (no dots), and two of the pairs were men (dots). In the upper right-hand corner we have 10 pairs in which the depressed individual was a low consumer of fish oil and the non-depressed individual was a high consumer of fish oil. The bottom left contains the pairs in which the non-depressed individuals were low consumers of fish oil and the depressed individual was not, and the bottom right contains pairs in which both case and control were high consumers of fish oil.

With the paired-data 2 × 2 table, we can now analyze these data to determine whether there is an association between fish oil consumption and depression, having taken account of potential non-comparability by sex in the design of the study by matching.

Analyzing Matched-Pair Data

In Figure 10.8 we summarize the matched-pair data that we outlined in Figure 10.7 by providing a sum of the number of pairs in each cell of the matched-pair 2 × 2 tables.

More generally, the 2 × 2 table of a matched-pair odds ratio is depicted in Figure 10.9.

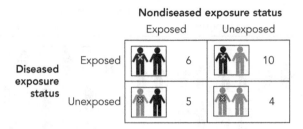

FIGURE 10.8 Summary of matched pairs in study on fish oil consumption and depression, matched on sex.

We have replaced the a, b, c, and d notation that we use for a traditional 2 × 2 table with e, f, g, and h to differentiate the matched-pair 2 × 2 from the unmatched 2 × 2.

What are the appropriate measures of association for case control matched-pair data? Given that we sampled these individuals based on disease status (i.e., we collected a sample of people with the outcome of interest, depression, and then collected a matched sampled of people without the outcome of interest), we know that the risk ratio and risk difference are inappropriate (see Chapter 6) and that an odds ratio is the best measure of association given this sampling design. However given that the data are matched, we need to use a matched-pair odds ratio:

$$\text{Matched-pair odds ratio} = \frac{f}{g}.$$

In a matched-pair odds ratio, only discordant pairs—those pairs in which one individual is exposed and the other is unexposed—in the 2 × 2 table contribute to the analysis.

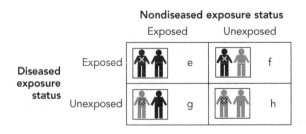

FIGURE 10.9 Matched-pair 2 × 2 table.

Thus, in our example of fish oil and depression, the matched-pair odds ratio is

$$\text{Odds ratio} = \frac{10}{5} = 2.0.$$

Thus, individuals with depression have 2.0 times the odds of low fish oil consumption compared with individuals who do not have depression, controlling for sex (as the data are matched on sex).

In Box 10.3 of the online material that accompanies Chapter 10, we detail how to estimate a confidence interval for a matched-pair odds ratio and provide an example of confidence interval estimation using the fish oil example.

Stratification

The two strategies that we have described thus far, randomization and matching, are strategies to control for non-comparability in the design stage of the study. Oftentimes we cannot randomize individuals because it is unethical or infeasible, and matching may or may not be an optimal strategy for all designs. For example, consider a large cohort study such as the Nurses' Health or Framingham study. These are ongoing cohorts of many thousands of individuals who are being regularly followed and tracked for a host of health outcomes and potential exposures. Through these studies we have learned a tremendous amount about the role of diet and other exposures on the development of chronic disease outcomes. To match these individuals based on potential non-comparability for just one research question would potentially limit our ability to monitor these other relationships. In general, matching is optimal when there is a specific hypothesis that is being tested, but it may not be the best choice when data are being collected on many exposure–outcome relationships simultaneously. Further, matching can be impractical when it limits our ability to find an appropriate control. In situations where both matching and randomization are not possible or optimal, another approach to control for non-comparability is when we are analyzing the data.

To control for non-comparability in the analysis stage of the study, the first and most fundamental point is that reliable, valid data must be collected on the potential variables that contribute to non-comparability. Variables that contribute to non-comparability between the exposed and the unexposed are often termed confounders in epidemiologic literature. Researchers must carefully and critically evaluate the potential factors that confound the associations of interest and include rigorous and careful measurement of these factors in the data collection stage. The ability to control for non-comparability in the analysis stage will only be as good as the quality of the measures of the variables contributing to non-comparability.

The next steps are to determine whether the variables meet several criteria for contributing to non-comparability in the data. Specifically, it is important to check whether the potential factor related to non-comparability is associated with the exposure and whether it is associated with the health indicator of interest. We did this in Chapter 9 in our example of alcohol consumption and esophageal cancer; smoking was both more common among heavy alcohol users and was associated with the development of esophageal cancer as well. We note that not all variables that are associated with the exposure and the health indicator of interest will contribute to non-comparability (see Box 10.4 in the online material that accompanies this chapter for more detail and examples); thus, these checks are necessary but insufficient to conclude that a particular factor is contributing to non-comparability.

Stratification removes the effects of a variable that is non-comparable between exposed and unexposed by limiting the variance on that outcome. We return to our example of alcohol consumption and esophageal cancer from Chapter 9. To control non-comparability through stratification, we examine the relation between alcohol consumption and esophageal cancer among two groups: those who smoke and those who do not. Among individuals who have never smoked a cigarette in their lives, for example, what is the relation between heavy alcohol consumption and esophageal cancer? Smoking cannot confound the effect estimate in this circumstance because no individuals in this subgroup have engaged in any smoking; thus, there is no variability in the restricted non-smoking sample on smoking prevalence. Similarly, among the group who are all smokers (presumably around the same duration and average amount) we also examine whether those who are heavy alcohol consumers are more likely to develop esophageal cancer. Again, smoking cannot confound the estimate because everyone in that subsample is a smoker.

We examine our study data for the relation between heavy alcohol consumption and esophageal cancer stratified by smoking status. First, in Figure 10.10, we examine the association among those who are nonsmokers.

Among the 22 nonsmokers, 6 are heavy alcohol consumers, whereas 16 are not. The conditional probability of esophageal cancer among those who are heavy alcohol consumers is 1/6, or 16.7%. The conditional probability of

	Health indicator present	Health indicator absent	Total N
Exposed	1	5	6
Unexposed	1	15	16
Total N	2	20	22

$$P(D|E+) = \frac{1}{6} = 0.167$$

$$P(D|E-) = \frac{1}{16} = 0.063$$

$$\text{Risk ratio} = \frac{0.167}{0.063} = 2.65 \; [95\% \; CI \; (0.20, 36.20)]$$

FIGURE 10.10 Association between heavy alcohol consumption and esophageal cancer among nonsmokers.

esophageal cancer among those who are not heavy alcohol consumers is 1/16 or 6.3%. Among nonsmokers, the risk ratio for heavy alcohol consumption on esophageal cancer is 2.65. Thus, there is an increased risk of esophageal cancer among heavy alcohol consumers, even in the subpopulation of individuals who do not smoke. However, the small cell sizes (reflecting the rarity of lung cancer among nonsmokers) would certainly raise concerns for us regarding inferring back to the population from these data.

We turn now to the smokers. In Figure 10.11, we examine the association between heavy alcohol consumption and esophageal cancer among the subgroup of individuals who smoke.

Among the 58 smokers, 31 of them are also heavy alcohol consumers. The conditional probability of esophageal cancer among those who are heavy alcohol consumers is 21/31, or 68%. The conditional probability of esophageal cancer among those who are not heavy alcohol consumers is 7/27 or 26%. Among smokers, the risk ratio for heavy alcohol consumption on esophageal cancer is 2.61. Thus, there is an increased risk of esophageal cancer among heavy alcohol consumers, even in the subpopulation of individuals who all smoke.

Note that without stratification on smoking, the association between alcohol consumption and esophageal cancer was 3.20 (see Figure 9.2). With

	Health indicator present	Health indicator absent	Total N
Exposed	21	10	31
Unexposed	7	20	27
Total N	28	30	58

$$P(D|E+) = \frac{21}{31} = 0.68$$

$$P(D|E-) = \frac{7}{27} = 0.26$$

$$\text{Risk ratio} = \frac{0.68}{0.26} = 2.61\ [95\%\ \text{CI}\ (1.32, 5.17)]$$

FIGURE 10.11 Association between heavy alcohol consumption and esophageal cancer among smokers.

stratification, the magnitude of the association decreased to ~2.6 among both smokers and nonsmokers. This indicates that there is evidence in the data that smoking is a source of non-comparability between the exposed and unexposed. Further, there remains an association between alcohol consumption and esophageal cancer that is independent of the effects of smoking on esophageal cancer.

In general, stratification of the data by a variable that contributes to non-comparability in the data will change the estimate of the association between the exposure and the health indicator. This change may result in an estimate that is closer to the null of no association, or further from the null of no association (see an example of this in the following section).

In summary, heavy alcohol consumption is associated with esophageal cancer both among a subpopulation of individuals who smoke and a subpopulation who do not smoke. Smoking cannot have any effect on the outcome within these subpopulations because there is no variance (i.e., all individuals within the subpopulation engage in the same amount of smoking behavior). By stratifying our analysis on a third variable that we believe is a cause of non-comparability, we can obtain estimates of the exposure–disease relation that are not confounded by that third variable, removing that source of non-comparability from the estimate of the association.

An Example Where Non-Comparability Suppresses the Effect

Thus far, our examples have exemplified non-comparability where the third variable of interest creates the appearance of an association that is larger than it should be. But non-comparability can work in the opposite direction as well. Non-comparability can mask an association that is really much larger than we see in our effect estimates. One example of this is the relation between cigarette smoking and depression. It has long been observed that the rate of depression is higher among cigarette smokers than among nonsmokers (Boden, Fergusson, & Horwood, 2010). Investigating whether there is a causal effect of smoking on depression is an important question, and a randomized trial is not possible given the many known adverse health consequences of smoking. Therefore, we need to sample individuals who smoke and do not smoke without randomization. However, we may want to think about how sex could be a potential source of non-comparability in this association. Men are more likely than women to be smokers, thus there will be a higher percentage of men in the smoker group than in the nonsmoker group. With regard to depression, however, men are less likely to experience depression compared with women; so there will be a smaller percentage of men in the depressed group than in the non-depressed group.

We see how this non-comparability of the association between smoking and depression by sex would manifest empirically.

Shown in Figure 10.12 are hypothetical data from a prospective cohort study on the relation between smoking and depression with each individual in the figure representing 10 people.

The population of interest is adults in the general population, and we collect a purposive sample of 80 individuals with no history of depression.

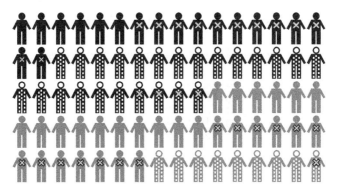

FIGURE 10.12 Studying the relation between smoking and depression.

We assess their smoking status and then follow them over 5 years to see how many individuals develop depression. Assume that no individuals were lost to follow-up. Those with dots are men and those without dots are women. First, we examine the overall association between smoking and the onset of depression, shown in Figure 10.13.

Thus, over 5 years, smokers had 1.034 times the risk of developing depression compared with nonsmokers, and 1.05 times the odds. The risk difference tells us that there is 1 excess case of depression per 100 persons who smoke compared to persons who do not smoke over the course of 5 years. But we must take account of sex before drawing conclusions from these data. To do this, in Figure 10.14, we first examine whether there is an association between smoking and sex as well as between depression and sex in these data.

	Health indicator present	Health indicator absent	Total N
Exposed	160	260	420
Unexposed	140	240	380
Total N	300	500	800

$$P(D|E+) = \frac{160}{420} = 0.38$$

$$P(D|E-) = \frac{140}{380} = 0.37$$

$$Risk\ ratio = \frac{0.38}{0.37} = 1.03\ [95\%\ CI(0.86, 1.24)]$$

$$Risk\ difference = 0.38 - 0.37 = 0.01\ [95\%\ CI(-0.05, 0.08)]$$

$$Odds\ ratio = \frac{\frac{160}{300}}{\frac{140}{300}}{\frac{260}{500}}{\frac{240}{500}} = \frac{160 * 240}{260 * 140} = 1.05\ [95\%\ CI\ (0.79, 1.41)]$$

FIGURE 10.13 Association between smoking and the development of depression.

	Smoker	Non-smoker	Total N
Male	+ = 240 200 40	+ = 90 80 10	330
Female	+ = 180 60 120	+ = 290 160 130	470
Total N	420	380	800

$$\text{Prevalence of smoking among men} = \frac{240}{240+90} = 0.73 = 73\%$$

$$\text{Prevalence of smoking among women} = \frac{180}{180+290} = 0.38 = 38\%$$

	Depressed	Not depressed	Total N
Male	+ = 50 40 10	+ = 280 200 80	330
Female	+ = 250 120 130	+ = 220 60 160	470
Total N	300	500	800

$$\text{Prevalence of depression among men} = \frac{50}{50+280} = 0.15 = 15\%$$

$$\text{Prevalence of depression among women} = \frac{250}{250+220} = 0.53 = 53\%$$

FIGURE 10.14 Determining whether sex is associated with smoking and depression.

We see that 73% of the men and 38% of the women are smokers; men are about 1.9 times more likely to smoke compared with women, 95% CI [1.66, 2.17]. Thus, we confirm in the data that men are more likely to be smokers than women. We also see that 15% of the men are depressed versus 53% of the women. Thus, women are about 3.51 times more likely to have depression compared with men, 95% CI [2.68, 4.59]. We can conclude that men are less likely to have depression compared with women.

Now we conduct a stratified analysis to examine the association between smoking and depression restricting only to the men (Figure 10.15) and then restricting only to the women (Figure 10.16). We focus on the risk ratio as the measure of association of interest. We return to this example in Chapter 11 when we discuss interaction and return to the measures of risk difference and the odds ratio.

We find that among men, those who smoke have 1.5 times the risk of depression compared to those who do not smoke, over 5 years. However, we note that the confidence interval is quite wide, suggesting that the range of underlying population values that would be consistent with sampling variability from these data are too wide to come to firm conclusions about the association between smoking and depression in these data.

Among women, those who smoke have 1.49 times the risk of depression compared with those who do not smoke.

Recall that when we did not stratify by sex, we found that smoking was not associated with depression. Once we stratify by gender, we see that smoking is associated with the development of depression. Thus, sex obscured the association between smoking and depression; and had we not controlled for sex,

	Health indicator present	Health indicator absent	Total N
Exposed	40	200	240
Unexposed	10	80	90
Total N	50	280	330

$$P(D|E+) = \frac{40}{240} = 0.17$$

$$P(D|E-) = \frac{10}{90} = 0.11$$

$$Risk\ ratio = \frac{0.17}{0.11} = 1.50 [95\%\ CI(0.78, 2.87)]$$

FIGURE 10.15 Smoking and depression among men.

	Health indicator present	Health indicator absent	Total N
Exposed	120	60	180
Unexposed	130	160	290
Total N	250	220	470

$$P(D|E+) = \frac{120}{180} = 0.67$$

$$P(D|E-) = \frac{130}{290} = 0.45$$

$$Risk\ ratio = \frac{0.67}{0.45} = 1.49\ [95\%\ CI(1.26, 1.75)]$$

FIGURE 10.16 Smoking and depression among women.

we would have concluded that there is no association between smoking and depression when in fact there is an association.

There are three key points underlying assessment of non-comparability through stratification. First, that careful and rigorous measurement of potential non-comparable variables is key to control for non-comparability in the data analysis stage of the study. Second, before stratification, one should always check that the potential non-comparable variables are associated with the exposure and associated with the outcome under study. Even if a variable is associated with the exposure and the outcome, however, it may not necessarily be a variable contributing to non-comparability. See more on this in Box 10.4 of the online material that accompanies this chapter. Finally, remember that if a variable is not associated with both exposure and outcome, then stratifying or otherwise controlling for that variable will not change the estimate of the effect of exposure on outcome.

Summary

In this chapter we have introduced three ways in which we can mitigate the problem of non-comparability in our studies. We can randomize the exposure, match individuals in the study on factors that contribute to non-comparability, or stratify the analysis on these factors and examine associations within strata. These are just three of many methods to reduce non-comparability in our studies. Non-comparability can become exceedingly complicated as factors that contributed to non-comparability change over time as the exposure changes over time, and when there are numerous factors contributing to non-comparability that interact in complex ways. By understanding the fundamental ways in which we control for non-comparability, we lay the foundations for understanding more complex data structures.

References

Boden, J. M., Fergusson, D. M., & Horwood, L. J. (2010). Cigarette smoking and depression: Tests of causal linkages using a longitudinal birth cohort. *British Journal of Psychiatry, 196*, 440–446.

Rossouw, J. E., Anderson, G. L., Prentice, R. L., LaCroix, A. Z., Kooperberg, C., Stefanick, M. L. . . . Writing Group for the Women's Health Initiative. (2002). Risks and benefits of estrogen plus progestin in healthy postmenopausal women: Principal results from the Women's Health Initiative randomized controlled trial. *Journal of the American Medical Association, 288*, 321–333.

11

When Do Causes Work Together?

IN OUR SEVEN-STEP approach to conducting an epidemiological study, we have progressed through the first five steps, including defining a population, the multiple ways to sample from a defined population, estimation of measures of disease occurrence and frequency from those samples, comparison of measures across groups, and assessment of the comparisons in our study for non-comparability.

Even when we have a well-defined and well-measured exposure and outcome, a well-designed study with minimal loss to follow-up and rigorous assessment of potential non-comparability, our work is not finished. We thus move to the sixth step in our seven-step approach, which entails assessing our data for evidence that causes may be working together. As we learned in Chapter 7, causes of disease rarely act in isolation. For nearly all health indicators that are of interest to public health, our exposures of interest are embedded in a host of other component causes that work together to activate the exposure's effect. In developing and testing hypotheses regarding the potential effects of an exposure on a health indicator, it is critical to conceptualize, measure, and assess the other component causes that may work in concert with the exposure of interest. When multiple component causes work together to produce a particular health indicator, we term this process interaction, as in the two component causes interact to cause a particular outcome. This frequently manifests in our data as an effect of an exposure on a health indictor (e.g., risk or rate ratio, risk or rate difference) varying across levels of another component cause. In this chapter, we discuss interaction conceptually from an epidemiologic point of view and discuss how we assess interaction in our data. We take special care to outline the differences between non-comparability and interaction. Interaction is often termed "effect measure modification" in other epidemiology textbooks and "moderation" in other disciplines; we consider these terms synonymous.

Introducing Interaction Conceptually: Back to Marble Jars

In Chapter 7, we described how the process of disease causation can be conceptualized as a collection of marbles. Each individual has a marble jar that, when filled with certain combinations of marbles, can initiate the disease process. In the population, there may be many different combinations of marbles that cause health indicators across populations. We review one example, considering a hypothetical disease in Farrlandia that we term *Epititis*. Figure 11.1 shows that there are two ways that Epititis is caused.

Some individuals in the population acquire Epititis because they have a family history of Epititis and are exposed to toxins in utero, each of which can be considered a component cause, or a marble in a marble jar. These two component causes together constitute a sufficient cause, and individuals who have both of them will get the disease. However, not all individuals with Epititis will have been exposed to family history and prenatal exposure; other individuals acquire Epititis because they have 20 pack-years of smoking, live in low-income neighborhoods, are male, and undergo stressful experiences in adulthood. These four component causes also form a sufficient cause that produces Epititis in some individuals. When marbles work together in the same marble jar to cause a health outcome, we say that they interact. That is, causes that interact are those in which both factors are necessary to cause disease through at least one sufficient cause.

Stepping back from health for a moment, consider by analogy what it takes for a sprinter to win a race. A sprinter has to have years of training to win a

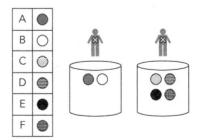

Sufficient cause 1
A = Family history
B = Exposure to toxins in utero

Sufficient cause 2
C = 20 pack-years of smoking
D = Neighborhood poverty
E = Male sex
F = Stressful experiences in adulthood

FIGURE 11.1 Causes of Epititis.

100-meter dash. But training alone may not be enough. She also needs to have properly tied running shoes and needs to react promptly to the starter's pistol to win the race. The weather may affect her performance, including wind and rain conditions. She has to properly stretch. She needs to have slept well the night before. Therefore, her extensive training alone will not get her to win the race. She also needs other component causes to work in concert with training for her to win. Similarly, most causes of disease work in concert with other causes—this is the case both for biological systems within individuals and for other causes external to the individual.

In our Figure 11.1 example, exposure to toxins in utero interacts with family history because they work together to produce Epititis. Similarly, smoking and neighborhood poverty, smoking and male gender, stressful experiences and smoking, and any other combination of these four exposures also interact to produce Epititis.

Interaction Versus Non-Comparability

Although male sex and family history are both component causes of Epititis in our example, they are in different marble jars and hence they do not interact. For us to say that two components interact, they need to work together within the same marble jar. However, the causes that do not work together (e.g., smoking and family history are both component causes but do not work together) may nonetheless still be associated. For example, those who are exposed to toxins in utero may be more likely to live in poor neighborhoods. If we were interested in the effect of exposure to toxins in utero on the development of Epititis in adulthood, we worry about the effect of poor neighborhoods in producing non-comparability across our study groups. There will be a greater proportion of individuals living in a poor neighborhood among those exposed to toxins in utero. Therefore, as we discussed in Chapter 10, we need to create comparability between those exposed to toxins and those unexposed to toxins on neighborhood poverty to estimate the causal effect of exposure to toxins in utero. That, however, is a different concept than interaction.

To illustrate the difference between the concepts of comparability and interaction, consider this question: Would family history of Epititis create non-comparability when we compare those exposed and unexposed to toxins in utero? Family history and in utero exposure are part of the same set of marbles that cause Epititis, that is, they are part of the same sufficient cause of Epititis. Therefore, if an individual is going to develop Epititis as a result of marble jar 1 (Figure 11.1), she or he will be exposed to both family history of Epititis and toxins in utero because these two component causes are both needed to complete marble jar 1. Therefore there is no variation in the relation between either of these two component causes (marbles) and the outcome (Epititis) when one or the other is present. If the individual only has one of these, that person will not develop Epititis through this sufficient causal pathway. Empirically, this means that we see the effect of one exposure (e.g., family history) varying across levels of the other potential component cause (e.g., toxins), and we can say that family history and toxins interact to produce disease.

In summary, when assessing the effect of in utero exposure to toxins on Epititis, we need to worry about the effects of living in a poor neighborhood, being male, having stressful experiences, and smoking a pack a day for 20 years as potential sources of non-comparability between exposed and unexposed. Family history, however, is part of the marble jar through which in utero exposure to toxins causes Epititis. It does not create non-comparability between exposed and unexposed but instead interacts with exposure to produce the disease. Importantly, this represents a different way in which we consider how to conceptualize a wide range of potential causes when designing and implementing epidemiologic studies. Although, as discussed in Chapters 8–10, we make substantial effort in epidemiology to make sure that sources of non-comparability are not alternative explanations for the observed association between the exposure of interest and the outcome, interactions are not alternative explanations. They are part of the explanation for the causal architecture that underlies the way in which the exposure of interest works to produce the outcome. We want to explain and report interaction.

In contrast, non-comparability arises when component causes that do not work together in the same marble jar are associated. Interaction arises when component causes are in the same marble jar and work together to produce a health indicator. The tricky part is, of course, that we, as epidemiologists, are not omniscient; and although we can carry out studies that show that particular marbles (e.g., family history, toxins, poor neighborhood, being male, stressful experiences, 20 pack-years of smoking) are associated with a particular health indicator (Epititis), we have no way of knowing with certainty whether causes act together in the same marble jar or whether they are in different marble jars. However, our data can give us strong signals regarding whether two exposures act together to produce the disease. In the rest of the chapter, we discuss how we interpret these signals.

Assessing Interaction in Data

In Chapter 7 we described how, if we were omnipotent, we could determine with certainty who will develop a health indicator—we could do this by measuring every component cause in every marble jar. Those who would inevitably get the disease would be those exposed to all component causes in a particular marble jar. If we knew all of those component causes, we would not need to use probability to describe risk of disease; we could determine with 100% accuracy who would get the disease and who would not. Those with all of the component causes in a marble jar would have 100% risk of disease; everyone else would have 0%. This is because all the component causes in a marble jar interact. This is an extreme example of how to assess for the presence of interaction in our data.

Although we rarely (if ever) know all of the marbles in a marble jar, the same concept applies when we are trying to measure interaction—we assess the risk of disease among those exposed to several factors at once compared to other groups. Then we examine whether those who have two (or more) exposures that are hypothesized to interact have a different risk of disease compared with those who have only one exposure or none of those exposures. We can spot interaction when the effect of an exposure on the outcome differs across levels of a second exposure.

For example, we are interested in whether consuming alcohol before driving is associated with risk of dying in a motor vehicle crash. We are also interested in the contribution that other factors may make to the risk of dying in a motor vehicle crash; for example, time of day when the driving occurs and whether the driver was wearing a seatbelt. Thus, there are two key research questions. First, does alcohol consumption prior to driving cause a greater risk of dying in a motor vehicle crash? Second, does alcohol consumption interact with time of day and/or seatbelt use in causing motor vehicle crashes? Understanding the answer to these questions can be quite informative about the conditions that lead to death in motor vehicle crashes. If, for example, alcohol consumption interacts with seatbelt use but does not interact with time of day, and if time of day is associated with risk of death as well as alcohol consumption, this would suggest that we had (at least) two sufficient causal pathways—one involving alcohol and seatbelt use together in one marble jar and one involving time of day (and potentially other component causes). This would highlight the need for efforts that target both causal pathways if we want to reduce deaths associated with motor vehicle crashes.

How would we answer these questions in the context of an epidemiologic study?

In Farrlandia, we select a representative sample of 10,000 individuals from the adult population and collect data on drivers, amount of alcohol consumed before driving, and whether they subsequently died in a motor vehicle crash. We also collect data on the time of day that the driving occurred (daylight vs. nighttime) and whether the driver was wearing a seatbelt. We stratify the data on alcohol consumption and risk of death by the two factors: seatbelt use and time of day (Figure 11.2). The x-axis shows the amount of alcohol consumed and the y-axis shows the risk of death.

What do these figures show us? First, we see that alcohol use is always associated with greater risk of death, supporting our hypothesis that alcohol use is potentially a component cause of death in motor vehicle crashes. But what about the other potential component causes?

Beginning with seatbelt use, we can see that among those who did not consume alcohol before driving, those who did not wear a seatbelt had a higher risk of dying in a crash (6%) than those who did wear a seatbelt (1%). We examine whether there is evidence in these data that indicate the effect of alcohol use on crash death varies by seatbelt use.

Among those who did not wear a seatbelt, the risk of dying in a crash was 10% among those who consumed alcohol prior to driving and 6% among those who did not consume alcohol prior to driving. The risk difference is thus

$$\text{Risk difference} = 0.10 - 0.06 = 0.04, 95\% \text{ CI } [0.03, 0.05].$$

There were 4 excess deaths per 100 drivers associated with alcohol consumption compared with no consumption.

Among those who did wear a seatbelt, the risk of dying in a crash was 5% among those who consumed alcohol prior to driving and 1% among those who did not consume alcohol prior to driving. The risk difference is thus

$$\text{Risk difference} = 0.05 - 0.01 = 0.04, 95\% \text{ CI } [0.03, 0.05].$$

Again, there were 4 excess deaths per 100 drivers associated with alcohol consumption compared with no consumption.

Thus, there is no difference in the risk difference between those who do and do not use a seatbelt, although using a seatbelt is associated itself with crash death. This indicates that seat belt use and alcohol use are part of different marble jars in our causal schematic and do not operate jointly to cause crash death.

(a) Seatbelt use

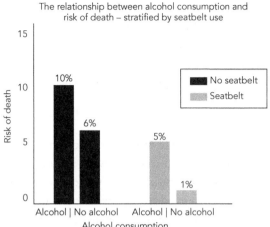

(b) Time of day

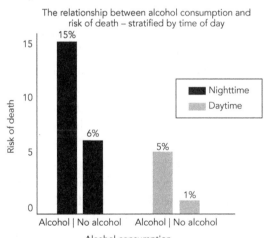

FIGURE 11.2 Stratifying alcohol consumption and risk of death by (a) seatbelt use and (b) time of day.

Now we assess the time of day in which the driving occurred. Similar to seatbelt use, we can see that, overall, there is a higher risk of crash death among drivers at night compared to during the day.

Among those who drove at night, the risk of dying in a crash was 15% among those who consumed alcohol prior to driving and 6% among those who did not consume alcohol prior to driving. The risk difference is thus

$$\text{Risk difference} = 0.15 - 0.06 = 0.09, \ 95\% \ \text{CI} \ [0.07, 0.11].$$

Among nighttime drivers, there were 9 excess deaths per 100 drivers associated with alcohol consumption compared with no consumption.

Among those who drove during the day, the risk of dying in a crash was 5% among those who consumed alcohol prior to driving and 1% among those who did not consume alcohol prior to driving. The risk difference is thus

$$\text{Risk difference} = 0.05 - 0.01 = 0.04, \ 95\% \ \text{CI} \ [0.03, 0.05].$$

indicating that among daytime drivers, there were 4 excess deaths per 100 drivers associated with alcohol consumption compared with no consumption.

The risk difference associated with alcohol consumption is 0.09 for nighttime drivers and 0.04 for daytime drivers. This indicates the presence of interaction—alcohol consumption increases the risk for death no matter the time of day, but consuming alcohol and driving at night is associated with an even higher risk of death than consuming alcohol and driving during the day.

In summary, we can examine the evidence for interaction in our data by comparing the magnitude of the association between exposure and disease across a third variable that we hypothesize to interact with the exposure of interest. If the measure of association differs across levels of the third variable, then there is evidence of interaction for that measure. If the measure of association does not differ across levels of the third variable, then there is no evidence of interaction between the third variable and the exposure of interest.

Interaction Across Scales

In the example of alcohol consumption and risk of motor vehicle crash, we assessed whether interaction is present by comparing risk differences across strata of seatbelt use and time of day. One uncomfortable fact of interaction, however, is that the presence of interaction depends on the measure of association that we are examining. We see why using an example.

We conduct a study in Farrlandia to investigate whether consumption of green tea is associated with reduced risk of stomach cancer. We are also interested in whether the association between green tea and stomach cancer varies by whether individuals have diets that are rich in smoked and cured food (consumption of smoked and cured foods is associated with a higher risk of stomach cancer; Fritz & Soos, 1980). We collect a purposive sample of 4,000 individuals without stomach cancer in Farrlandia. We purposively collect 1,000 individuals in each of four groups: 1,000 individuals who drink green tea and do not eat smoked/cured foods; 1,000 who drink green tea and eat smoked/cured foods; 1,000 who do not drink green tea but eat smoked/cured foods; and 1,000 who do not drink green tea and do not eat smoked/cured foods. All individuals are follow forward in time for 20 years to determine which individuals develop stomach cancer over the study time period. There is no loss to follow-up.

In Figure 11.3 are the 2 × 2 tables describing the study findings. Individuals who drink green tea are colored black, and individuals who consume smoked/cured foods are dotted.

These data indicate that among those who do not eat smoked/cured foods, green tea consumption is associated with 0.50 times the risk, 95% CI [0.70, 1.46], and 0.50 times the odds, 95% CI [0.70, 1.46], of stomach cancer compared with those who do not consume green tea. Among those who consume smoked/cured foods, green tea consumption is associated with 0.80 times the risk, 95% CI [0.45, 1.43], and 0.80 times the odds, 95% CI [0.44, 1.44], of stomach cancer compared with those who do not consume green tea.

Thus, based on the risk ratio and the odds ratio, green tea consumption appears to have a stronger protective effect among those who do not consume smoked/cured meats than among those who do consume such food because 0.5 is a stronger effect compared with 0.8. That is, a risk ratio of 0.5 signifies that exposure decreases the risk of stomach cancer compared by about 50%, compared with the unexposed; a risk ratio of 0.8 signifies that exposure decreases the risk of stomach cancer compared by about 20%, with the unexposed. Based on the risk and odds ratios, we might then conclude that there is evidence of interaction between green tea and smoked/cured foods.

However, the risk differences across the two strata are exactly the same, at −0.005 in both strata. The risk difference of −0.005 indicates that green tea consumption is associated with 5 fewer cases of stomach cancer for every 1,000 individuals who consume green tea compared with those who do not, regardless of whether an individual consumes smoked/cured foods or not.

Among those who do not eat smoked/cured foods

	Health indicator present	Health indicator absent	Total N
Exposed	5	995	1000
Unexposed	10	990	1000
Total N	15	1985	2000

$$P(D|E+) = \frac{5}{1000} = 0.005$$

$$P(D|E-) = \frac{10}{1000} = 0.01$$

$$\text{Risk ratio} = \frac{0.005}{0.01} = 0.50 \ [95\% \ CI \ (0.17, 1.46)]$$

$$\text{Risk difference} = 0.005 - 0.01 = -0.005 \ [95\% \ CI(-0.01, 0.00)]$$

$$Odds \ ratio = \frac{\dfrac{\frac{5}{15}}{\frac{10}{15}}}{\dfrac{\frac{995}{1985}}{\frac{990}{1985}}} = \frac{5*990}{995*10} = 0.50 \ [95\% \ CI \ (0.17, 1.46)]$$

Among those who eat smoked/cured foods

	Health indicator present	Health indicator absent	Total N
Exposed	20	980	1000
Unexposed	25	975	1000
Total N	45	1955	2000

$$P(D|E+) = \frac{20}{1000} = 0.02$$

$$P(D|E-) = \frac{25}{1000} = 0.025$$

FIGURE 11.3 Association between green tea consumption and cancer, stratified by consumption of smoked/cured foods.

$$\text{Risk ratio} = \frac{0.02}{0.025} = 0.80 \ [95\% \ \text{CI} \ (0.45, 1.43)]$$

$$\text{Risk difference} = 0.02 - 0.025 = -0.005 \ [95\% \ \text{CI}(-0.02, 0.01)]$$

$$\text{Odds ratio} = \frac{\dfrac{\dfrac{20}{45}}{\dfrac{25}{45}}}{\dfrac{\dfrac{980}{1955}}{\dfrac{975}{1955}}} = \frac{20*975}{980*25} = 0.80 \ [95\% \ \text{CI} \ (0.44, 1.44)]$$

FIGURE 11.3 Continued

Based on the risk difference, we might conclude that there is no evidence of interaction between green tea and smoked/cured foods.

This example illustrates a central concept in the assessment of interaction. Namely, that interaction is dependent on whether we use a ratio measure to assess associations or a difference measure. In fact, when two exposures both have an association with an outcome, there will always be interaction on at least one scale but possibly not both.

So what do we conclude? Is there interaction between green tea and smoked/cured food consumption or not? The answer has substantial public health implications. If there is interaction, then encouraging people to drink green tea will reduce stomach cancer to a greater extent among those who do not eat smoked/cured foods. Unless we can promote both messages effectively, we are not able to maximally effect public health. If there is no interaction, then we should focus our public health dollars on promoting green tea consumption alone. To understand how to interpret findings when there is interaction only on one scale but not the other, we need to understand additivity and multiplicativity.

Additivity, Multiplicativity, and Interaction

We can mathematically understand why interaction is scale dependent using a simple example.

We assess interaction on two scales: additive and multiplicative.

If two exposures do not interact on an additive scale, then the risk of disease among those exposed to both is the sum of the risk of disease given exposure to one factor plus the risk of disease given exposure to the other factor. If two exposures do not interact on a multiplicative scale, then the risk of disease among those exposed to both is the product of the risk of disease given exposure to one factor multiplied by the risk of disease given exposure to the other factor.

For example, consider a hypothetical disease A with the following risks:

Example 1:

Among those exposed to both X and Y (R_{11}): 10%

Among those exposed to X but not Y (R_{10}): 6%

Among those exposed to Y but not X (R_{01}): 5%

Among those exposed to neither X nor Y (R_{00}): 1%

We can assess whether there is evidence that X and Y interact on an additive scale by using the following formula:

$$R_{11} - R_{00} = R_{10} - R_{00} + R_{01} - R_{00},$$

where R_{11} is the risk of disease among those exposed to both X and Y (10%), R_{10} is the risk of disease among those exposed to X but not Y (6%), R_{01} is the risk of disease among those exposed to Y but not X (5%), and R_{00} is the risk of disease among those exposed to neither X nor Y. Thus, our example yields

$$(6 - 1) + (5 - 1) = (10 - 1).$$

In this example, the risk of disease among those exposed to both X and Y is equal to the sum of the risk associated with exposure to X alone, plus Y alone, subtracting the baseline risk (risk among those exposed to neither X nor Y) from each estimate for mathematical accuracy.

Thus, there is no evidence of additive interaction. There is, however evidence of multiplicative interaction. To assess for multiplicative interaction, we can use the following formula:

$$(R_{11}/R_{00}) = (R_{10}/R_{00}) * (R_{01}/R_{00}).$$

If this equation is satisfied in our data, then there is no evidence of multiplicative interaction. However, in our data we observe that the produce of the (R_{10}/R_{00}) and (R_{01}/R_{00}) is greater than (R_{11}/R_{00}):

$$(6/1) * (5/1) = 30.$$

Because 30 > 10, there is evidence of multiplicative interaction. The observed risk ratio is 10.0 (10/1), much less than the expected 30.0 [(6/1)*(5/1)]. Thus, the risk ratios do something less than multiply, indicative of an interaction between X and Y on the multiplicative scale.

We consider a second example, a hypothetical disease B with the following risks:

Example 2:

Among those exposed to both X and Y: 30%

Among those exposed to X but not Y: 6%

Among those exposed to Y but not X: 5%

Among those exposed to neither X nor Y: 1%

Using our two formulae as described previously, we first assess additive interaction:

$$\text{Does } R_{11} - R_{00} = R_{10} - R_{00} + R_{01} - R_{00} ?$$

No, it does not, because $(6 - 1) + (5 - 1) \neq 30 - 1$. Thus, there is evidence of additive interaction.

Second, we assess multiplicative interaction:

$$\text{Does } \left(R_{11} / R_{00} \right) = \left(R_{10} / R_{00} \right) * \left(R_{01} / R_{00} \right)?$$

Yes, it does, because $(6/1) * (5/1) = (30/1)$. Thus, there is no evidence of multiplicative interaction.

To summarize, in Example 1, there is no evidence of additive interaction because the risks associated with either exposure alone sum to the risk associated with both. Yet there is evidence of multiplicative interaction. In Example 2, there is no evidence of multiplicative interaction because the risks associated with either exposure alone multiply to the risk associated with both. Yet there is evidence of additive interaction. Thus, there is interaction present in both of these examples, and simultaneously, interaction absent in both of these examples. It all depends on the scale that we are assessing.

This is uncomfortable because in epidemiology, as in all science, we prefer to have firm answers to straightforward questions. When we ask, "Does X interact with E to cause disease D," the unsatisfying answer is, "Well, it depends on what measure of association you are assessing." Given the public health importance of questions regarding interaction, this answer is problematic.

Substantial scholarship in epidemiological methods has shown that, in general, additive interaction (e.g., interaction of risk differences or rate differences) corresponds more closely to our understanding of the causal concepts described at the beginning of this chapter (Rothman, Greenland, & Walker, 1980; VanderWeele & Robins, 2007), that is, suggesting two (or more) component causes coexisting within the same sufficient cause. Therefore, when two factors are causal partners in the same sufficient cause, the resulting measures of association will depart from additivity but not necessarily from multiplicativity. In general we recommend, as do a growing number of epidemiologists, that interaction—or the search for marbles that co-occur in the same marble jar—be assessed on an additive scale. Despite this, statistical interaction on the multiplicative scale can often also be demonstrated. Whereas statistical interaction on the multiplicative scale is a form of interaction when interaction is defined as non-independence of effect estimates, we focus here on additive interaction because it more closely corresponds to our understanding of causal processes.

Assessing Additive Interaction With Ratio Measures

We have now seen that interaction arises when there are two (or more) component causes of the same sufficient cause influencing the outcome of interest. We look for evidence of interaction in our data by assessing whether the measure of association between exposure and outcome differs across levels of a third variable. We have also seen that the evidence for interaction will be dependent on the measure of association used and suggest that additive interaction is the scale that most closely corresponds to our causal frameworks. We illustrated an example of testing for additive interaction using risk differences. We could also demonstrate additive interaction by assessing whether rate differences vary across levels of a third variable.

Often times, however, we may not be able to estimate risk or rate differences. For example, when our study design is to collect individuals with and without a health indicator of interest (case control study), we cannot estimate population parameters for risks and rates directly because our study design dictates the number of diseased and non-diseased participants. We have learned, in Chapter 6, that the odds ratio is an appropriate measure of association for these types of study designs. We provide an overview of testing for additive interaction using odds ratio measures in Box 11.1 of the online material that accompanies this chapter and provide an overview of special considerations when using odds ratios to assess interaction in Box 11.2.

Accounting for Random Variation in Assessments of Interaction

As with any measure of association, measures of interaction (whether comparison of risk differences or use of interaction contrasts with ratio measures) can arise due to chance in the sampling process. That is, by chance we may collect a sample in which there is a large proportion of individuals with disease in a certain subgroup. Therefore, creating confidence intervals around interaction measures is of considerable importance. The development of statistical methods for assessment of interaction is not as advanced as other statistical fields, and there remains some lack of consensus about the best practices for creating confidence intervals for assessments of additive interaction. Due to the complexity of some of these measures, they are outside the scope of an introductory textbook, but we refer interested readers to the following sources: Hosmer and Lemeshow (1992) and Richardson and Kaufman (2009).

Summary

Interaction occurs when two causes are both components of the same sufficient cause. When two causes interact, we mean epidemiologically that at least some individuals become diseased through a sufficient cause that includes both component causes (plus, potentially, others). We can think of interaction as one thinks of the factors that need to work together for a sprinter to win her race—she needs to be well trained, well rested, have proper running shoes, and react to the starting pistol to win, among other considerations. Similarly, many other factors often need to be present for a certain exposure to cause disease. The factors that cause the sprinter to win the race, together, interact. In our data, we can observe interaction when the measure of association for an exposure and an outcome varies across levels of a third variable. The observation of interaction is complicated, however, by the fact that the appearance of interaction may depend on the scale we are considering (additive or multiplicative). In epidemiology, we are principally concerned with interaction on the additive scale. Therefore, variation in the risk difference across levels of a third variable, or interaction contrast ratios for ratio measures (see online compendium material for Chapter 11), are the most appropriate means of assessing interaction in our data. Interaction is conceptually quite distinct from non-comparability in that interaction does not create spurious association or mask true associations; rather, interaction illuminates causal pathways and synergies across data sources that enrich our hypotheses and further elucidate causal processes.

References

Fritz, W., & Soos, K. (1980). Smoked food and cancer. *Bibliotheca Nutritio et Dieta, 29,* 57–64.

Hosmer, D. W., & Lemeshow, S. (1992). Confidence interval estimation of interaction. *Epidemiology, 3,* 452–456.

Richardson, D. B., & Kaufman, J. S. (2009). Estimation of the relative excess risk due to interaction and associated confidence bounds. *American Journal of Epidemiology, 169,* 756–760.

Rothman, K. J., Greenland, S., & Walker, A. M. (1980). Concepts of interaction. *American Journal of Epidemiology, 112,* 467–470.

VanderWeele, T. J., & Robins, J. M. (2007). Four types of effect modification: A classification based on directed acyclic graphs. *Epidemiology, 18,* 561–568.

12

Do the Results Matter
Beyond the Study Sample?

WE HAVE ARRIVED at the last step of the seven-step approach outlined in Chapter 1 for conducting epidemiologic studies. Given what we have learned up to this point, we can now assess the extent to which the results of our study are applicable in populations outside of the underlying population base of our particular study. We now understand how to sample from a defined population, count cases, estimate associations, rigorously test those associations for validity by mitigating non-comparability, and assess the evidence for causes working together. And yet our work is still not finished. In any study, we need to think through the characteristics of our population of interest and determine how robust the study findings might be across populations with similar or different characteristics. The process of evaluating our findings beyond the study sample is often termed generalizability, or synonymously, external validity. In this chapter, we formalize a framework for conceptualizing the factors that make a study finding externally valid beyond the population of interest. To do so, we first briefly review several different stages of validity to explain how external validity fits in with what we have covered so far.

Stages of Validity

Before we can understand external validity, it is important to consider the precursors necessary to even begin to consider whether a study result is valid beyond the study sample. Fundamentally, an association cannot be valid beyond the study sample unless it is valid within the study sample. Here we draw on a framework articulated by Shadish, Cook, and Campbell (2002) to introduce four types of validity that are important to consider when interpreting findings from a study. We can conceptualize these types of validity as building on each other, each being necessary before the next can be achieved.

The first is measurement validity, which in epidemiologic applications can be conceptualized as the accuracy and precision of our measurements of exposure, disease, potential sources of non-comparability, and potential causal partners of the exposure. The central question for measurement validity is whether we have actually measured what we intended to measure. If we have not measured what we meant to measure, then the conclusions we can draw from our data are minimal if anything.

The second is statistical conclusion validity. Once we know we have robust measures, and we document an association, we should be concerned with whether the association observed is due to chance. We have noted throughout this book that we use confidence intervals around our estimates of association to describe the role of sampling variability in generating the results we obtain in the study. Thus, statistical conclusion validity is ruling out with a reasonable degree of confidence the potential that our results arose by chance in the sampling process from an underlying population of interest.

Once we are sufficiently confident that our result is not due to poor measurement, or to chance in the sampling process, the third type of validity to consider is internal validity. Internal validity refers to the assessment of non-comparability between exposed and unexposed being an unlikely explanation for our study results. That is, a result that is internally valid is a causal result: It is the causal effect of the exposure on the outcome. We discussed internal validity in more detail in Chapters 8 through 10. Without internal validity, it is meaningless to apply the association documented in the sample to other populations.

Once we have established measurement, statistical conclusion, and internal validity, we can then begin to consider external validity.

Introduction to External Validity

The applicability of study findings beyond the study sample is typically termed the study's external validity. We have come to conceptualize this as whether, and to whom, the results from our study matter. We begin the discussion of external validity by recalling that we start an epidemiologic study by first identifying a population of interest and then sampling from that population. In some circumstances, we may take a random sample of the population, thereby maximizing the representativeness of the sample for characteristics of the population. In other circumstances, we may take a purposive sample of the population, selecting individuals based on specific eligibility criteria in a way that may not be representative of that population but rather to maximize the comparability between exposed and unexposed.

Regardless of how the sample was obtained, the underlying population of interest for the sample result should be clearly delineated, and the sample result should be reflective of the underlying association in that population of interest (within bounds of sampling variability). For example, our underlying population of interest may be all adult women, 18 years or older, in the United States; or all persons born in the United Kingdom in 1990. The reason why the population of interest should be clearly articulated is, in part, so that the external validity of the study results can be clearly articulated.

Understanding External Validity Through Prevalence of Component Causes

Central to our understanding of external validity is an understanding of the prevalence and distribution of component causes of the health indicator of interest across populations.

We first elaborate on this concept through a simplified example. We are interested in whether exposure to ambient air pollution causes lung cancer and believe that smoking is a component cause of ambient air pollution (i.e., part of a network of causes that together interact to cause lung cancer in at least some people). That is, for our example, ambient air pollution will cause lung cancer, but only among individuals who smoke, reflecting the co-occurrence of ambient air pollution and smoking within the same sufficient cause. Similarly, smoking will cause lung cancer but only among individuals who are exposed to ambient air pollution. Individuals can also acquire disease through an unrelated set of causes; for the example, we term the people who acquire lung cancer not through smoking and ambient air pollution the "genetically determined" group and assume that a portion of people in our sample will acquire lung cancer because of genetic vulnerability, regardless of exposure to ambient air pollution or smoking. Therefore, genetic determination represents another sufficient cause of lung cancer.

Now, suppose we have two populations, each consisting of 20 people. Our study data are shown in Figure 12.1. Out of the 20, 10 people in both studies are exposed to ambient air pollution. The study samples are comparable with respect to the distribution of genetic determinism, as shown in the summary

Black = Exposed to air pollution
Dots = Genetically determined
Hat = Smoker

Population 1

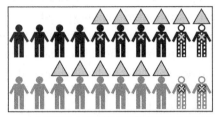

	Exposed to pollution N = 10 (Black)	Unexposed to pollution N = 10 (Gray)
Genetically determined (Dots)	2	2
Smokers (Hat)	6	6

Population 2

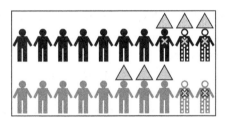

	Exposed to pollution N = 10 (Black)	Unexposed to pollution N = 10 (Gray)
Genetically determined (Dots)	2	2
Smokers (Hat)	3	3

FIGURE 12.1 Two study populations in which we are assessing the influence of ambient air pollution on lung cancer risk.

table; thus there is no confounding and perfect internal validity. That is, 2 people in both Population 1 and Population 2 acquire disease through genetic determinism, and genetic determinism is equally distributed between exposed and unexposed in both populations. The main difference between the two populations is the prevalence of smoking. In Population 1, 6 people are smokers, both in the exposed and in the unexposed to ambient air pollution. In Population 2, 3 people are smokers, both in the exposed and the unexposed to ambient air pollution. What result would we obtain if we calculate the effect of ambient air pollution on lung cancer?

We calculate the risk difference associated with ambient air pollution in Population 1. Among those exposed, 6 develop the disease, for a risk of 60%. Among those unexposed, 2 develop the disease, for a risk of 20%. Thus, the risk difference is 40%, suggesting that 40 cases of lung cancer are associated with ambient air pollution per 100 exposed. Notice that this is a causal effect because we have perfect comparability between exposed and unexposed regarding genetic determinism.

Now we calculate the risk difference associated with ambient air pollution in Population 2. Among those exposed, 3 develop the disease, for a risk of 30%. Among those unexposed, 2 develop the disease, for a risk of 20%. Thus, the risk difference is 10%, suggesting that 10 cases of lung cancer are associated with ambient air pollution per 100 exposed. Similar to Population 1, this is a causal effect because again, we have perfect comparability between the exposed and unexposed on genetic determinism.

We have two studies that asked the question, "What is the causal effect of ambient air pollution on lung cancer?" Both are internally valid studies because the exposed and unexposed are comparable on genetic determinism. However, in the first study, of Population 1, the causal effect is a risk difference of 40%; and the causal effect in the second study, of Population 2, is a risk difference of 10%.

Why do these two causal effects differ? Note, critically, that the prevalence of people exposed to ambient air pollution is the same in both studies, as is the prevalence of genetic determinism. The reason that these two causal effects diverge is because there was a different prevalence of smoking between the two populations.

This should remind the reader of our discussion of interaction in Chapter 11. As we covered in that chapter, when two causes interact, the measure of association for the effect of one cause on the outcome will differ across levels of the second cause. Because the two causal effect estimates differ and there is no non-comparability, we can conclude that ambient air pollution and smoking are causal partners within the same sufficient cause, and the prevalence of one of them (smoking in this case) influences the causal effect of the other (ambient air pollution) on the outcome (lung cancer).

Extending our example, we expect that the causal effect of ambient air pollution on lung cancer would differ across any population in which the prevalence of smoking also differs. There is not one causal effect for all populations; the causal effect is dependent on the prevalence of smoking in each population.

This is true of almost all epidemiologic effect measures when assessing the impact of potential causes that are neither necessary nor sufficient to cause disease in populations. The magnitude of an association, whether measured on the risk difference, risk ratio, rate, or odds scale, will depend on the prevalence of the component causes of the exposure of interest. Therefore, and here is the heart of the matter, the result from one study will be externally valid to populations in which the distribution of component causes of the exposure is similar to the study sample.

Before we move on from this point, we note that differing prevalence of causal partners across populations is a critical way in which a result may not be externally valid, but it is not the only way in which results may not be externally valid. We present differing causal partners as a key way in which we can begin to draw conclusions beyond our study sample and populations of interest, as an introduction to the process of external validity. We refer the reader to more advanced epidemiologic writing to elaborate on the other ways in which results may or may not be externally valid (Hernan & VanderWeele, 2011).

Cause, Causal Effect, Study Design, and External Validity

We now understand that the particular magnitude of association in any particular study is dependent on the component causes of the exposure of interest within the population that serves as the base of the study sample. The magnitude of the association will, then, be applicable beyond the study to the extent that the distribution of causal partners of the exposure is similar in other populations.

In the physical and natural sciences, scientists are often interested in identifying general truths about the world—absolute theorems that are always true—such as gravitational forces and the components of the Krebs cycle. Similarly, in epidemiology, it is often our goal to discover general truths about the causes of human disease. If we want to identify something as a cause of disease, should it be a cause absolutely and in all types of populations? The answer to that question requires us to conceptualize causes not in isolation but within a network of interacting causes.

Within an individual case of a health indicator, a cause is a factor that was necessary for that disease to occur in that person at that time. Because most causes are insufficient and unnecessary in isolation, a single cause catalyzes the onset of disease in an individual within a network of embodied component causes that interact with the exposure of interest. But in epidemiology and population health we do not study individuals, we study populations; therefore, we study not causes but causal effects. That is, we study the association between those who embody the cause (the exposed) and those who do not (the unexposed). A causal effect in a population is context specific and dependent on the prevalence of component causes. A cause that produces a tremendous amount of disease or other adverse health outcomes in one population may be negligible with respect to population health in another population. Alternatively, a cause may produce relatively or absolutely similar amounts of adverse health outcomes across populations given stability of the distribution of causal partners. If we care about what matters most to population health, then understanding a cause in the context of its causal partners needs to be central to our theorizing, our design, and our analysis, for it is only through this endeavor that we can understand the distribution of causes and their effects within and across populations.

In summary, the concept of identifying causes of health indicators is central to epidemiology, and the causes that we identify help us to shed light on the scientific process of disease occurrence in humans. There are many causes of adverse health, and each of these causes will produce adverse health in any population with a non-zero prevalence of the component causes that interact with the causes to produce the disease. But the magnitude of a causal effect, or the size of the association between the cause and the outcome, is context-specific, tied to the particular characteristics of a place and time insofar as the prevalence of the causal partners varies across populations and time.

It is important to note that changing distributions of causal partners across populations and across time is not inevitable. For example, most studies of smoking and lung cancer, across many populations, have estimated strong and relatively consistent effects for the size of the association between smoking and lung cancer (Lee, Forey, & Coombs, 2012). Thus, there is general consistency in the magnitude of the association between smoking and lung cancer, regardless of the population studied, and whether it is a representative sample. This tells us something important, namely, that the prevalence of the causal partners of smoking is relatively consistent across many types of populations. For other potential causes, the result may not be as consistent but is no less causal than is the relationship between smoking and lung cancer.

External Validity Versus Internal Validity: A Trade-Off

We noted at the beginning of this chapter that internal validity (the lack of non-comparability between the exposed and unexposed) is a prerequisite to external validity. To achieve internal validity, we often need to design a study with a very narrow population of interest in mind. We do so, of course, to minimize non-comparability. For example, we may be more likely to have comparable exposed versus unexposed groups if our sample was comprised only of 42-year-old women living in Massachusetts, where there might be less intra-sample heterogeneity on a whole range of factors than if our sample included women and men, of all ages, from multiple states. We select unexposed persons that are comparable on all causes of disease to the exposed persons, but the resulting sample may not be reflective of a broader swath of the population beyond the underlying population of interest from which the exposed and unexposed persons arose. For example, randomized trials often have strict and numerous criteria for a potential subject to be recruited into the study. Randomized trials are often designed to recruit only individuals with good potential for adherence to the study protocol and with a low degree of co-occurring medical problems. The effect estimate obtained from such a trial, because we randomized the exposure and hence minimized non-comparability, is likely to have strong internal validity. But the more narrow our sample becomes due to strict inclusion and exclusion criteria to achieve internal validity, the less external validity it may have if there are causal partners of the exposure that have differing prevalence in the study sample compared with other types of population groups (Greenhouse, Kaizar, Kelleher, Seltman, & Gardner, 2008).

Thus, we make a trade-off. In building the scientific argument for a causal effect of an exposure on an outcome, we first select a study design and conduct a study to rigorously assess the internal validity of our causal question. Once we have established that the exposure has a causal effect with a very narrow and very select population, we then expand the causal question to ask how often, among whom, and under what conditions the exposure has a causal effect. Therefore, we might conduct a randomized trial and obtain an estimate of a causal effect that does not apply to any population outside of the underlying population that was recruited into the study. A representative sample, on the other hand, may yield an excellent sample in terms of the applicability of the study findings to a broad population of interest, but it can be more difficult than other designs to achieve rigorous causal inference through control of non-comparability.

In Boxes 12.1 and 12.2 of the online material that accompanies this chapter, we present examples of hypothetical studies to discuss the problems and solutions for judging external validity from epidemiologic studies.

Summary

In summary, we have now concluded discussion of the seven foundational steps through which we conduct epidemiologic studies. We identify a population of interest; create measures of exposures and health indictors; take a sample of that population; count cases as they arise and compare the occurrence of adverse health among exposure groups; assess the extent to which these associations may be causal; assess the potential causal partners of exposures of interest; and finally, evaluate the extent to which the prevalence of potential causal partners differs between the population that gave rise to the study sample and other populations for which we might use the study results and evidence to intervene. Through these steps we can conduct an epidemiology of consequence and rigorously understand the complex process through which adverse health arises in populations and ultimately embeds in individuals.

References

Greenhouse, J. B., Kaizar, E. E., Kelleher, K., Seltman, H., & Gardner W. (2008). Generalizing from clinical trial data: A case study. The risk of suicidality among pediatric antidepressant users. *Statistics in Medicine, 27*, 1801–1813.

Hernan, M. A., & VanderWeele, T. J. (2011). Compound treatments and transportability of causal inference. *Epidemiology, 22*, 368–377.

Lee, P. N., Forey, B. A., & Coombs, K. J. (2012). Systematic review with meta-analysis of the epidemiologic evidence in the 1900s relating smoking to lung cancer. *BioMed Center Cancer, 12*, 385.

Shadish, W. R., Cook, T. D., & Campbell, D. T. (2002). *Experimental and quasi-experimental designs for generalized causal inference.* Boston: Houghton Mifflin.

13

How Do We Identify Disease
Early to Minimize Its
Consequences?

AS WE HAVE discussed throughout the book, we design epidemiologic studies
to estimate the occurrence and frequency of disease in populations of interest
and to identify causes of disease and other health indicators so that we may do
something about these causes, that is, so that we may intervene and prevent
disease. Epidemiology also makes another contribution to the prevention of
disease. We develop and assess tools that can identify early signs of specific
diseases and syndromes and, therefore, can predict who will develop adverse
health conditions. The early detection of individuals who are at risk for the
development of specific health states, or the identification of individuals who
are in the early stages of a particular disease, is called screening. Although
we do not include screening in our seven steps for an epidemiology of consequence, screening remains a foundational method in epidemiology that is
critical for the introductory student to understand. In this chapter we cover
the basics of screening for disease, including when to screen, how to screen,
and how to evaluate results from studies that assess the efficacy of screening
programs in improving population health.

What Is Screening?

Screening is the process by which we use a test to determine whether an individual likely has a particular health indicator or not, or is likely to develop a
particular health indicator or not. Screening tests are typically probabilistic—
they give us information about whether the disease is likely to be present; but
follow-up examinations and tests are often necessary before we can make a
definitive diagnosis.

Most of us have undergone routine screening during the course of our encounters with the health care system. For example, most women receive regular screening tests beginning in young adulthood for cervical cancer (known as the "Pap smear"). Physicians assess blood pressure and cholesterol as screening tools for the development of cardiovascular disease. Screening tools extend beyond illness and disease, however. For example, women who use a home pregnancy test are screening for the presence of an embryo or fetus in their uterus. All of these tests rely on data that has shown that the test is able to detect people who have the health indicator under investigation, and sometimes equally, if not more important, the ability of the test to correctly identify those without the health indicator.

A screening test typically assesses the presence of an underlying marker that is believed to be associated with the health indicator of interest. Individuals who are above a certain threshold on the marker are sent for additional testing, biopsy, or other confirmatory diagnosis. There are two central considerations when evaluating a screening test. First, how good is the test at identifying cases and non-cases; and second, is it appropriate to introduce the screening test into clinical practice?

How Good Is the Screening Test at Identifying Cases and Non-Cases?

The first step in evaluating whether screening for a particular health indicator is appropriate is to determine the validity and predictive capability of the test itself. To determine if a screening test is going to be useful, we have to compare it to an established test that is considered the gold standard for diagnosis. That is, to evaluate a screening test, we need to have information on whether an individual actually has, to the best of our ability to determine, the disease or health indicator of interest. We then evaluate the screening test using four related parameters: (a) sensitivity, (b) specificity, (c) positive predictive value, and (d) negative predictive value. In describing these parameters, we use binary states for both the screening test and the gold-standard diagnosis (i.e., an individual either screens positive or negative and either has a diagnosis or no diagnosis for the health indicator), although of course we recognize that many health indicators exist on a continuum.

Table 13.1 is a summary of the relevant parameters. As shown in the table, each individual falls into one of four categories. Among those who actually have the health indicator under investigation, individuals can either screen positive or negative. Those who screen positive are true positives, and those

Table 13.1 Screening Parameters

	Diagnosis Positive	Diagnosis Negative	Screening Parameter
Screen positive	True positive (TP)	False positive (FP)	$PPV = \dfrac{TP}{TP + FP}$
Screen negative	False negative (FN)	True negative (TN)	$NPV = \dfrac{TN}{TN + FN}$
Screening parameter	Sensitivity $= \dfrac{TP}{TP + FN}$	Specificity $= \dfrac{TN}{TN + FP}$	

Note. PPV = positive predictive value; NPV = negative predictive value.

who screen negative are false negatives (i.e., they screen negative even though they do have the health indicator). Among those who do not have the health indicator under investigation, individuals can also screen positive or negative. Those who screen negative are true negatives, and those who screen positive are false positives (i.e., they screen positive even though they do not have the health indicator). Using these four categories, we can in turn estimate the four key parameters of interest. If screening tests were perfect, there would be no false positives or false negatives. However, screening tests are rarely perfect. That is, having a particular screening marker usually does not mean one definitely will have a health indicator, but that one is more likely than not to have the health indicator, and vice versa. In the language we introduced in Chapter 7, we would say that screening tests are probabilistic rather than deterministic.

To demonstrate the principles of assessing a screening test, we consider a hypothetical scenario from Farrlandia. Public health professionals are worried about the high rates of prostate cancer among Farrlandian men. There is promise, however, in a new test that characterizes the level of an antigen in the blood demonstrated to be associated with prostate cancer. The test is inexpensive and requires only a blood specimen. We want to consider whether we should encourage all men to be tested for prostate cancer with the new screening tool. To make our recommendation, we first collect some data. We sample 240 men with confirmed incident diagnoses of prostate cancer, and 2,500 men who are confirmed to be free of prostate cancer. We measure their level of the antigen. Our data are shown in Figure 13.1.

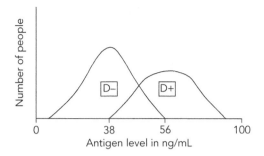

FIGURE 13.1 Distribution of the antigen among those with prostate cancer (D+) and without prostate cancer (D-) in Farrlandia.

We can see from Figure 13.1 that the mean level of the antigen is higher among those with prostate cancer compared with those without prostate cancer, but that the distributions of the antigen overlap to some degree. Specifically, there are both diseased and nondiseased persons with levels of antigen between ~38 and 56 ng/mL. This overlap is common in the markers that we use to screen for health indicators; that is, whereas there are some levels that denote individuals who are clearly diseased and some levels that denote individuals who are clearly free of disease, there is a certain range of values for which the disease status of individuals will be uncertain. It is in this uncertain range that we typically declare a cutoff, above which we label individuals as screening positive and below which we label individuals as screening negative. The chosen cutoff will have implications for the performance of the screening test.

Sensitivity and Specificity

We have already introduced sensitivity and specificity in Chapter 3 when we discussed the validity of a measure compared with a gold standard. The same concept applies here; we are assessing the validity of the screening tool in establishing the presence of the health indicator compared with a gold standard. With sensitivity and specificity, we want to know whether those with the health indicator are correctly identified by the screening test as having the health indicator (sensitivity) and whether those without the health indicator are correctly identified by the screening test as not having the health indicator (specificity).

For our screening test, we need to decide on a value of the antigen above which we label men as screening positive and send them for more invasive diagnostic testing. The lowest value on the antigen distribution of men with

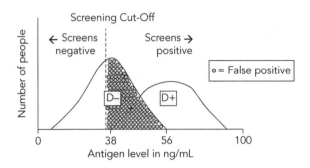

FIGURE 13.2 Distribution of the antigen among those with prostate cancer (D+) and without prostate cancer (D-)—with screening cutoff of 38 ng/mL.

prostate cancer is 38 ng/mL. We begin by assigning 38 ng/mL as our cutoff score. Figure 13.2 shows the distributions of the antigen, now with a vertical line marking the cutoff score.

With our cutoff score established, we can now create a 2 × 2 table to display the quantitative results of the screening test performance (Table 13.2).

We can then evaluate these results to understand the value of the screening test.

Among Those With the Disease, What Proportion Does Our Screening Test Correctly Identify?

That is, among those with prostate cancer, what proportion would the test, at a 38 ng/mL cutoff, detect? This is the sensitivity of the test.

$$\text{Sensitivity} = \frac{\text{True positive}}{\text{True positive} + \text{False negative}};$$

$$\text{Sensitivity} = \frac{240}{240 + 0} = 1.0 \text{ or } 100\%.$$

Table 13.2 Screening Test Results Labeling Those With ≥38 ng/mL as Screened Positive

	Diagnosis Positive	Diagnosis Negative	**Total**
Screen positive	240	971	1,211
Screen negative	0	1,529	1,529
Total	240	2,500	2,740

With a cutoff of 38 ng/mL, we have a test with 100% sensitivity. This indicates that among those with prostate cancer, the test captures all cases. There are no false negatives (individuals who have the disease but do not screen positive in our test). We can see this clearly in Figure 13.2. Note that no individual who is on the curve on the right, that is, the curve of those with disease, will be missed with a screen at the 38 ng/mL cutoff. This then becomes a perfectly sensitive test—a positive screen always identifies those with disease. But, as we can also see from Figure 13.2, just because the test is highly sensitive it does not mean it is the best cutoff—we first also need to examine the test's specificity.

Among Those Without Disease, What Proportion Does Our Screening Test Correctly Identify as Disease Free?

That is, among those without prostate cancer, what proportion would the test, at a 38 ng/mL cutoff, correctly identify as not having prostate cancer? This is the specificity of the test.

$$\text{Specificity} = \frac{\text{True negative}}{\text{True negative} + \text{False positive}};$$

$$\text{Specificity} = \frac{1529}{1529 + 971} = 0.612 \text{ or } 61.2\%.$$

Thus, our screening test only classifies 61.2% of men without prostate cancer as not having prostate cancer. The remaining 38.8% are false positive cases (individuals who do not have the disease but screen positive in our test).

In our attempt to capture all cases of prostate cancer using the 38 ng/mL cutoff, we necessarily declare ~39% of men without prostate cancer as potential cases, sending them for more invasive procedures. The procedure for definitive diagnosis may have risks, high cost, and produce anxiety in patients who are told that they may have prostate cancer. Thus, screening may be neither cost-effective nor acceptable if ~39% of individuals without the disease will be sent for invasive testing and diagnosis.

In summary, in this example, the test cutoff is very sensitive, in that all those who have the health indicator will be captured by the screening test, but not very specific because many individuals who do not have the health indicator will screen positive. High sensitivity/low specificity tests are quite common in practice. Consider, for example, the current guideline that primary care physicians query patients about whether they engaged in at least one episode of heavy drinking in the past year as a screening tool for identifying individuals with an alcohol disorder (Willenbring, Massey, Gardner, 2009). Almost all individuals with an alcohol disorder will have engaged in at least one episode of heavy drinking in the past year, but many individuals without an alcohol disorder may have engaged in one or more heavy drinking episodes as well. Thus, the test is sensitive, but not specific.

Positive and Negative Predictive Value

Once we have the sensitivity and the specificity of the test, we next ask how well our screening test predicts who has the health indicator and who does not. We evaluate this through positive and negative predictive values.

Among Those Who Screen Positive, What Proportion Actually Has the Disease?

Here we are asking, among those who have an antigen level at or above 38 ng/mL, what proportion has prostate cancer? This is the positive predictive value (PPV) of the test for this sample.

$$PPV = \frac{\text{True positive}}{\text{True positive} + \text{False positive}};$$

$$PPV = \frac{(240)}{(240 + 971)} = 0.198 \text{ or } 19.8\%.$$

About one fifth of the men who screen positive on our test have prostate cancer, leaving about 80% of men screening positive falsely. We note that as an individual being screened, the positive predictive value is perhaps the most intuitive and important metric to be aware of. If a Farrlandian goes to his health provider and is told that he has screened positive for prostate cancer, he will, almost certainly, feel quite anxious and worried. But, if the Farrlandian were to ask, "What is the positive predictive value of this test?," he would quickly realize that, in fact, he is more likely than not to be just fine—only one fifth of all men who screen positive have prostate cancer after all! This is worth remembering for all of us whenever we receive a screening test.

Among Those Who Screen Negative, What Proportion Actually Do Not Have the Disease?

Here we are asking, among those who have an antigen level below 38 ng/mL, what proportion is free of prostate cancer? This is the negative predictive value (NPV) of the test for this sample.

$$NPV = \frac{\text{True negative}}{\text{True negative} + \text{False negative}};$$

$$NPV = \frac{(146)}{(146+0)} = 1.0 \text{ or } 100\%.$$

Our test has perfect negative predictive value. That is, among those who are negative on the screening test, we can be perfectly confident that none of those individuals actually have the disease. Given that our test has no false negatives, this should not be a surprise.

In summary, we assess sensitivity and specificity to understand the proportion of those with and without the health indicator who are correctly categorized. We assess PPV and NPV to understand the proportion of positively screened and negatively screened individuals that have and do not have the health indicator, respectively. In our example, we were able to correctly categorize all individuals with the health indicator using our screening test, but we had a high rate of false positives, leading to lower specificity and lower PPV than is ideal.

Changing Screening Cutoffs: Effects on Screening Test Parameters

Our hypothetical screening test for prostate cancer set a cutoff of 38 ng/mL on an antigen that is related to prostate cancer. Our resulting screening test had perfect sensitivity and negative predictive value, but the high percentage of false positives led to low specificity and positive predictive value. We now change the cutoff on the screening test to determine the effects on screening parameters. Suppose, now, that we increase the cutoff to 45 ng/mL. That is, we consider individuals positive on the screening test if the level of antigen is 45 ng/mL or above. Using the same data, we observe the results in Table 13.3.

Table 13.3 Screening Test Results Labeling Those With ≥ 45 ng/mL as Screened Positive

	Diagnosis Positive	Diagnosis Negative	Total
Screen ositive	217	424	641
Screen negative	23	2,076	2,099
Total	240	2,500	2,740

$$\text{Sensitivity} : \frac{217}{217+23} = 0.904 \text{ or } 90.4\%$$

$$\text{Specificity} : \frac{2076}{2076+424} = 0.830 \text{ or } 83.0\%$$

$$\text{PPV} : \frac{217}{217+424} = 0.339 \text{ or } 33.9\%$$

$$\text{NPV} : \frac{2076}{2076+23} = 0.989 \text{ or } 98.9\%$$

We now have sensitivity and specificity of 90.4% and 83%, respectively. Compared with our original cutoff of ≥38 ng/mL, our sensitivity decreased, but specificity increased substantially, from 61.2% to 83%. Why did sensitivity decrease? By increasing the screening cutoff, some individuals who have prostate cancer will now screen negative on our test, leading to false negatives. As we increase the cutoff for positivity on a screening test, the number of individuals with the health indicator of interest who screen negative will likely increase, leading to lower sensitivity. However, we gain specificity, because fewer individuals without the health indicator will screen positive.

The positive predictive value of the test also increased substantially when we raised the cutoff, from 19.8% to 33.9%. The PPV increased due to the decrease in false positives; that is, when there are fewer false positives, the probability that an individual who screens positive will actually have the health indicator will increase.

In Figure 13.3 we show visually how changing screening cutoffs will influence the proportion of false positives and false negatives.

As we see on Panel 1 of the graph, those from the disease negative distribution who are above the screening cutoff will be labeled as positive, thus forming the false positive group. In Panel 1, we set the cutoff low enough that there is no one from the disease positive distribution who is below the screening

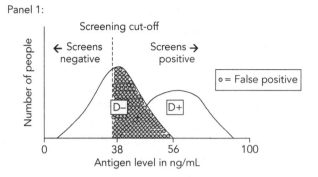

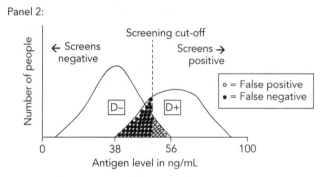

FIGURE 13.3 Distribution of the antigen among those with prostate cancer and without prostate cancer—impact of changing screening cutoffs.

cutoff, leading to no false negatives. In Panel 2, the cutoff is moved to a higher antigen level. We can see that there are now fewer individuals from the disease negative distribution who screen positive, thus leading to fewer false positives. Now, however, there are individuals from the disease positive distribution who have an antigen level below the cut point, leading to false negatives.

In summary, an increase in the screening cutoff will decrease sensitivity and NPV because the number of false negatives will increase. An increase in the screening cutoff will increase specificity and PPV because the number of false positives will decrease. The reverse of each is true if we decrease the screening cutoff; the number of false negatives will decrease, and the number of false positives will increase.

How Do We Decide on the Appropriate Cutoff?

We have shown through the preceding examples that the screening parameters of sensitivity, specificity, PPV, and NPV will change based on the cutoff selected for a screening test. How, then, do we select the appropriate cutoff?

Fundamentally, any cut-off decision will be associated with certain limitations and trade-offs. Determining cutoffs involves, as we have noted here, trade-offs, and the right cutoff is a matter of which we value most: false positives or false negatives. There are some ways of thinking about this that can help guide us in our selection.

First, we need to consider the potential ramifications of false positives versus false negatives. If we have false negatives on our screening test, then individuals could potentially leave the health facility unaware that they have a health problem. In the case of infectious diseases such as HIV, for example, maintaining a low rate of false negatives is critical, because individuals could unknowingly communicate disease to others. We thus might be willing to tolerate a higher rate of false positivity to achieve a low rate of false negativity. On the other hand, there may be health indicators for which a low rate of false positivity is preferred. If the subsequent diagnostic test involves invasive and expensive procedures (e.g., biopsy of a potentially cancerous site), we may be willing to tolerate a higher rate of false negativity for a low level of false positivity. Tests with high rates of false negativity are typically done on a routine basis to optimize disease detection (see Box 13.1 in the online material that accompanies this chapter for an example of such a test, the Pap smear for cervical cancer detection).

Second, there are empiric guidelines for optimizing screening cutoffs including receiver operating characteristic (ROC) curves. These are outside the scope of an introductory textbook, but interested readers are encouraged to learn more about ROC curves through several excellent texts including Beck and Shultz (1986) and Zou, Liu, & Bandos (2012).

Third, an increasingly common approach is to use a two-stage screening test, first screening individuals using a test with high sensitivity and then following up with a test with high specificity. In Box 13.2 in the online material that accompanies this chapter, we describe two-stage screening and provide a quantitative example.

Positive Predictive Value, Negative Predictive Value, and Disease Prevalence

We demonstrated in the previous section that PPV increased and NPV decreased when false positives are decreased and false negatives increased, respectively. But screening cutoffs are also influenced by an additional parameter, which is the overall prevalence of the health indicator in the population that is being screened.

To understand this principle, consider the following scenario. Using our antigen screening test with a cutoff of 45 ng/mL, we screen two separate samples for prostate cancer. The first sample is comprised of 1,500 men with a family history of prostate cancer who are older than 60 years of age. The second is a sample of 1,500 men of age 40 to 60 with no family history. The results based on each of these two samples are shown in Table 13.4.

First, we examine sensitivity and specificity. In both samples, sensitivity and specificity are 90% and 83%, respectively. However, PPV and NPV differ across the samples. In the sample of men over age 60 with a family history of prostate cancer, 72.7% of those who screen positive for prostate cancer actually have prostate cancer. In the sample of men aged 40 to 60 with no family history, only 3.4% of those who screen positive actually have prostate cancer. Whereas PPV is thus much higher in the first sample, the NPV is somewhat lower.

Why does PPV change so much in the two samples, even when sensitivity and specificity remain the same? PPV is dependent on the prevalence of the health indicator in the population that is being screened. As the prevalence increases, the probability that any individual who screens positive will be a true case increases because the overall probability of being a true case is also increasing. Conversely, the probability of being a true negative case decreases as the prevalence increases because the overall probability of not being a case is also decreasing. Sensitivity and specificity are not directly influenced by prevalence because for these parameters we look among those who have the health indicator versus those who do not.

In summary, PPV and NPV are dependent on prevalence, and PPV increases as the prevalence of disease increases. Because PPV will improve as prevalence increases, it is important to identify groups at higher risk of the development of the health indicator of interest for screening.

This concept is not simply of academic interest, and it came to bear in the controversial decision to change the recommended age to begin breast cancer screening (mammography) from 40 to 50 (Marmot et al., 2013). Because the incidence of breast cancer is low from age 40 to 49, it has been argued that the PPV of mammography is too low to justify the risks associated with follow-up testing for those who screen positive. That is, most women who screen positive on mammography between age 40 and 49 will be false positive; thus it has been suggested that there is little value to screening during that age range. However, this recommendation was not extended to women age 40 to 49 with a family history of breast cancer or other factors that increase risk. These women are at higher risk for breast cancer in the 40–49 age range; thus, the

Table 13.4 Screening for Prostate Cancer in Two Samples

Sample 1. Men Over 60 Years of Age With a Family History of Prostate Cancer

	Diagnosis Positive	Diagnosis Negative	Total
Screen positive	452	170	622
Screen negative	48	830	878
Total	500	1,000	1,500

$$\text{Sensitivity}: \frac{452}{452+48} = 0.904 \text{ or } 90.4\%$$

$$\text{Specificity}: \frac{830}{830+170} = 0.830 \text{ or } 83\%$$

$$\text{PPV}: \frac{452}{452+170} = 0.727 \text{ or } 72.7\%$$

$$\text{NPV}: \frac{830}{830+48} = 0.945 \text{ or } 94.5\%$$

Sample 2. Men Between 40 and 60 With No Family History of Prostate Cancer

	Diagnosis Positive	Diagnosis Negative	Total
Screen positive	9	253	262
Screen negative	1	1,237	1,238
Total	10	1,490	1,500

$$\text{Sensitivity}: \frac{9}{9+1} = 0.9 \text{ or } 90\%$$

$$\text{Specificity}: \frac{1237}{1237+253} = 0.830 \text{ or } 83\%$$

$$\text{PPV}: \frac{9}{9+253} = 0.034 \text{ or } 3.4\%$$

$$\text{NPV}: \frac{1237}{1237+1} = 0.999 \text{ or } 99.9\%$$

PPV of mammography would be sufficient for these women to justify the cost and risk of screening.

From Screening Test to Screening Program: Should We Introduce a Screening Test Into the Population?

Even if we have a screening test with high sensitivity and specificity, there are several considerations we must evaluate before introducing a screening test in the population. Screening is not necessarily cost-effective or health effective either for individuals or for communities. Screening tests are often expensive, and those who screen positive may need to undergo subsequent invasive testing for diagnostic purposes, which incurs additional expense and may involve risk to the patient. Therefore, introduction of a screening tool into a population needs to be carefully considered, and numerous rubrics for understanding when a screening tool is appropriate for introduction into the population have been developed (Hulka, 1988; Miller, 2012). We highlight several of these considerations in the following.

First among the considerations is its potential population health impact. Universal screening, for example, should be considered for health indicators that have substantial impact on population health as opposed to rare conditions for which the cost of screening many people to detect one case would be large.

Second, in deciding whether a screening program for a health indicator is appropriate, it is also critical to consider what is known about the natural history and progression of the health indicator of interest. Screening may be considered when there is a sufficiently long period of time between the biological onset of disease and the appearance of signs and symptoms of the disease and the disease is detectable during this period (e.g., through a biological or a radiographic marker). Therefore, this creates an opportunity for screening where we could detect the presence of the disease earlier than it would otherwise come to clinical attention.

Third, and critically, introducing a screening test into medical practice is appropriate only when there is an available treatment for the disease for which early detection would substantially improve the lives of those affected. Put another way, if we develop a screening test that picks up a disease a year earlier than its symptoms might have revealed it, but we cannot do anything for that disease anyway, there is little point to incurring the individual, and societal, costs of screening.

In summary, screening should be considered when the health indicator of interest is an important determinant of population health, when there is a substantially long phase in the natural history of the health indicator in which it can be detected before signs and symptoms appear, and when screening and early disease detection and treatment can result in improvement in the course of the disease. A good screening test, for example, the Pap test for cervical cancer, does all of this. Cervical cancer, without early screening and detection, is a significant contributor to the burden of disease among women throughout the world. However, early signs of the cancer are visible at the cellular level; and the Pap test takes a small cervical cellular sample that allows detection of the cancer at very early stages, when it is treatable. The Pap test has dramatically reduced the burden of cervical cancer through much of the world (Wright, 2007). Interestingly, cervical cancer provides a textbook example of epidemiology in action in more ways than simply screening. More recent developments in the field have included the identification—through breakthrough epidemiologic studies (Walboomers et al., 1999)—of human papillomavirus (HPV) that are precursors of cervical cancer and new vaccines, now widespread in adolescents, are preventing the onset of cervical cancer and changing the face of the disease worldwide. More detail on this is provided in Box 13.1 of the online material that accompanies this chapter.

There are other considerations that come into play in evaluating the utility of a particular screening test, such as costs to individuals and society of screening or not. We leave those considerations to other higher level epidemiology or population health science books.

How Do We Evaluate Whether a Screening Program Is Effective at Reducing Morbidity and Mortality?

Once we have a screening test with acceptable sensitivity and specificity, and we have identified eligibility criteria for a population to be screened that maximizes the positive predictive value of the test, we then need to ensure that screening actually has an impact on the population in terms of improving disease-related outcomes and lengthening life.

That is, a good screening test will identify individuals at risk for or with the health indicator of interest earlier than the absence of screening. However, without effective prevention and treatment tools for the health indicator, there is no purpose of early identification of individuals with the health indicator. Thus, once the validity of a screening test has been established, next the effectiveness of a screening program in reducing morbidity and mortality must be established.

How would such a study be conducted? We explicate these concepts using examples from cancer. Based on the principles of study design that we have learned thus far, we know that we need to compare cancer-related outcomes among a group that is screened for cancer with the outcome experience of a group that did not receive screening. We need to assess the groups for comparability of other causes of the study outcomes, through randomization, matching, or stratification. If screening has a beneficial effect on morbidity and mortality, the outcomes—including length of life—should be longer in the screened group compared with the non-screened group.

There are, however, two central complications that are particular to screening that complicate our evaluation of whether a screening test effectively reduces disease burden by comparing a group that is screened to a group that is not screened. We discuss these here.

Detection Based on Screening Is More Likely to Find Slow-Growing Tumors Compared With Detection Based on Symptoms

Shown in Figure 13.4 is the cancer experience of 20 individuals in Farrlandia across a 40-year period. The individual with an "X" indicates the onset of cancer, and the "X" without a corresponding individual indicates death (either from the cancer or from some other cause). We assume for this example that there is no remission or recovery from this cancer.

As is clear from the figure, there is variation in the duration of the cancer experience, with some cancers having a long duration during which an individual may die from an unrelated cause, and some cancers having a quite short duration.

Now, imagine that we screened these individuals for cancer at Year 10, shown in Figure 13.5.

Screening at a single time point is conceptually similar to estimating the prevalence of cancer at that time point. We get a snapshot of cancer in the one-time screening. Thus, it should not be a surprise, given what we know about prevalence (see Chapter 5), that the cancer cases that are more likely to be detected in the screening are those of long duration that are perhaps slow-growing tumors. This raises two problems.

The first problem is that it is possible these slow-growing tumors may not eventually cause death or disability in those affected. Remember that the

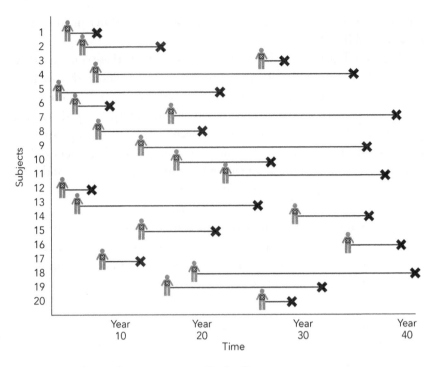

FIGURE 13.4 Cancer duration among 20 Farrlandians across 40 years.

purpose of screening is to detect cases before they are symptomatic and likely to come to clinical attention. It is possible that asymptomatic cancers will never become symptomatic and that they may not end up being the cause of death. For example, autopsy studies of men in old age suggest that the prevalence of asymptomatic prostate cancer is very high (Haas, Delongchamps, Brawley, Wang, & de la Roza, 2008); detecting asymptomatic prostate cancer and aggressively treating it may be ineffectual if the men would never have experienced symptoms of the cancer and eventually die of another cause. Unfortunately, it is difficult to predict which tumors will become symptomatic and which ones will not; and screening picks up cancers that may or may not be clinically relevant to an individual's life. This of course introduces problems with the net value of the screening test. Aside from the potential extra cost that we incur by screening for cancers we do not need to screen for, this also introduces morbidity (and potential mortality) to those screened. That is, if we are screening old men for cancers that will not harm them, we are subjecting them to treatments that may be more dangerous than the disease. There is no easy way to deal with this problem, and it is a consideration that

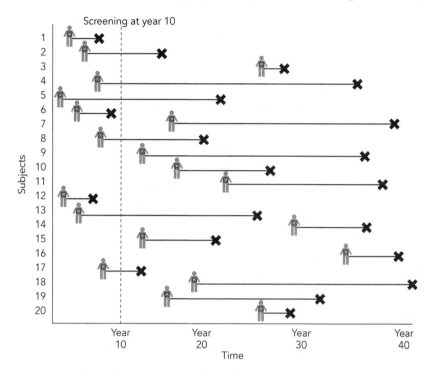

FIGURE 13.5 Cancer duration among 20 Farrlandians across 40 years, with screening at 10 years.

must be balanced when recommending whether a screening test should be implemented widely in a population.

The second problem is that the cancers that were detected by screening will tend to be less aggressive and include many that would never cause symptoms or death if left undetected. Thus, case fatality rate (proportion who die among those with cancer at any given time) among the screened will be lower than among the non-screened, but not because the screening itself lengthened the life of the individual. This will render a biased estimate of the causal impact of screening on morbidity and mortality and is referred to as length bias. There are no explicit methods to counteract length-time bias (because we cannot see into the future to know which cancers detected by screening will eventually become symptomatic). The possibility of length bias should also be acknowledged, and factored in, when evaluating the efficacy of a screening program. Epidemiology textbooks focused on screening provide more detail about how we deal with these challenges in practice (Nasca & Pastides, 2007).

Detection Based on Screening Provides Extra Lead Time to the Screened Group Even in the Absence of an Effect of Screening on Mortality

Even if screening has no effect on length of life or other potential cancer-related outcomes, a simple comparison of length of life between a group in which cancers are detected early from screening and a group in which cancers are detected when they become symptomatic may appear to show a benefit. To understand why, consider the example in Figure 13.6.

Person 1's cancer was detected through screening, whereas Person 2's cancer was detected due to the appearance of symptoms. The two individuals have the same time from cancer onset to death, indicating that the early detection of cancer in Person 1 did not cause her to live any longer than if she had not been screened. Yet the time from cancer detection to death is longer in Person 1 compared with Person 2, simply because her cancer was detected earlier (with no subsequent improvement in length of life). The time between detection of cancer from screening and detection of cancer through symptoms is termed the lead time afforded by the screening test. Comparison of length of life in two groups, one of which had lead time due to early disease

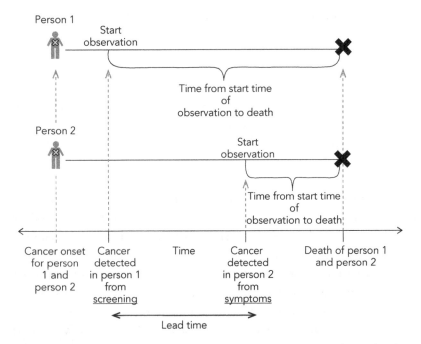

FIGURE 13.6 Length of life for two individuals with cancer; one cancer detected with screening, the other cancer detected from symptoms.

detection, will always show a benefit in the screened group, even if the early detection of the cancer did not actually lengthen the life of the individual. Thus, survival times between screened groups and non-screened groups must be carefully compared so that the lead time afforded by screening is not interpreted as a benefit of screening for length of life.

The difference in observation time between a group that is screened and a group that is not is thus a source of non-comparability between groups. As we know, if there are sources of non-comparability between groups, inference from a study can be compromised. Thus, the solution to the problem of differing observation times between groups is to create comparability with respect to observation time. An appropriately designed evaluation of a screening program compares survival time between screened and non-screened groups with the same start time. We show an example of this in Figure 13.7.

The two individuals now have the same start time of observation, which is independent of the appearance of symptoms of cancer. Now we see that the time from the start of observation to death is the same in the individual who was screened and the individual who was not screened, indicating that that there is no association between screening and length of life. This type of

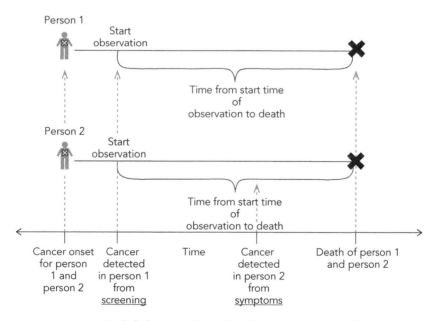

FIGURE 13.7 Length of life for two individuals with cancer showing no effect of screening on time to death; start time for observation follow-up equivalent between individuals.

design, where two groups are compared from the same start point of observation time, is common in randomized trials of screening tools.

Finally, we examine the individuals in Figure 13.8. Similar to the last two figures, there are two individuals, one of whom was engaged in screening and one of whom was not. Observation start time is invariant between the two individuals. Now we see that the time from the start of observation to death is shorter for the individual who was not screened compared with the individual who was screened. If this pattern is demonstrated in the average time from observation start time to death across groups who were screened and not screened, this would demonstrate evidence that early detection through screening has a benefit in terms of mortality.

Summary

Screening for health indicators is an integral part of improving population health, both by predicting who will develop a specific health indicator and by detecting these health indicators among those in the early stages. Screening tests need to be studied for validity by assessing sensitivity and specificity

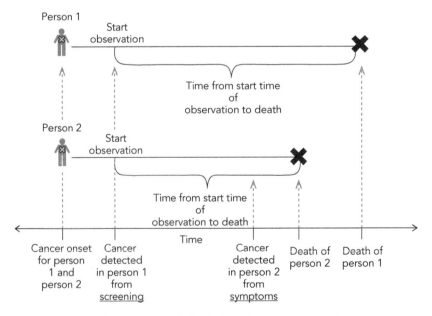

FIGURE 13.8 Length of life for two individuals with cancer showing a longer time to death among the screened compared with the unscreened individual; start time for observation follow-up equivalent between individuals.

compared with a gold standard. There is often a trade-off between sensitivity and specificity, and the decision about which parameter to maximize will depend on the specific characteristics of the health indicator of interest. The predictive value of a screening test will be maximized in a population with a high prevalence of the health indicator of interest. Once there is a valid and predictive screening test available, the value of a screening program will depend on a number of parameters. Screening programs should be cost-effective and minimally invasive. Most important, there must be available and effective treatment for the health indicator once cases are detected through the screening test. Evaluation of screening programs must contend with two important sources of non-comparability between screened and non-screened groups. First, cases that are detected by screening may be cases that would never have come to clinical attention; thus, the potential for over-treatment should be considered. Second, the start times of observation need to be comparable between screened and non-screened groups, otherwise the lead time afforded to the screened group may result in non-comparability and the appearance that the screening lengthened survival time.

References

Beck, J. R., & Shultz, E. K. (1986). The use of relative operating characteristic (ROC) curves in test performance evaluation. *Archives of Pathology & Laboratory Medicine, 110*, 13–20.

Haas, G. P., Delongchamps, N., Brawley, O. W., Wang, C. Y., & de la Roza, G. (2008). The worldwide epidemiology of prostate cancer: Perspectives from autopsy studies. *Canadian Journal of Urology, 15*, 3866–3871.

Hulka, B. S. (1988). Cancer screening. Degrees of proof and practical application. *Cancer, 62*(Suppl. 8), 1776–1780.

Marmot, M. G., Altman, D. G., Cameron, D. A., Dewar, J. A., Thompson, S. G., & Wilcox, M. (2013). The benefits and harms of breast cancer screening: An independent review. *British Journal of Cancer, 108*, 2205–2240.

Miller, A. B. (Ed.). (2012). *Epidemiologic studies in cancer prevention and screening.* New York: Springer.

Nasca, P. C., & Pastides, H. (Eds.). (2007). *Fundamentals of cancer epidemiology* (2nd ed.). Sudbury, MA: Jones & Bartlett.

Walboomers, J. M., Jacobs, M. V., Manos, M. M., Bosch, F. X., Kummer, J. A., Shah, K. V., . . . Munoz, N. (1999). Human papillomavirus is a necessary cause of invasive cervical cancer worldwide. *The Journal of Pathology, 189*, 12–19.

Willenbring, M. L., Massey, S. H., & Gardner, M. B. (2009). Helping patients who drink too much: An evidence-based guide for primary care clinicians. *American Family Physician, 80*, 44–50.

Wright TC. Cervical cancer screening in the 21st century: is it time to retire the PAP smear? *Clin Obstet Gynecol*, 2007.

Zou, K. H., Liu, A. & Bandos, A. (2012). *Statistical evaluation of diagnostic performance: Topics in ROC analysis.* Boca Raton, FL: CRC Press.

14

Conclusion: Epidemiology and What Matters Most

IN CHAPTER 1 WE defined epidemiology as the science of understanding the distribution and determinants of health and disease in populations so that we may intervene and improve public health. In this book, we have provided an overview of the process through which epidemiologic studies are designed, measures of exposure and health indicators are developed, and some basics of how data are analyzed. In this concluding chapter, we offer a few thoughts about the latter part of our charge as epidemiologists—to intervene to improve the public's health. In considering studies that aim to improve population health we do not mean to limit ourselves only to epidemiologic studies of specific interventions, but rather, we intend a fuller remit: an intent to conduct epidemiologic studies that have clear implications and consequences for the improvement of the public's health.

Epidemiologic studies provide the data that inform the science of population health. Our studies identify causes of health indicators and help us understand how these causes are distributed in populations. It is worth considering, however, the research questions that we ask and the way in which we conceptualize epidemiologic studies within a broad, global context that places questions about how we may improve population health and where our work can have the largest impact squarely in the forefront. We argue that epidemiology has a foundational responsibility to attempt to make a demonstrable impact on population health. We advocate, therefore, a consequentialist view toward epidemiologic research questions (Galea, 2013), one that focuses attention on outcomes of our research in terms of quantifiable benefits for human health. In other words, students and practitioners should engage in an epidemiology of consequence that asks critical questions not about whether exposure X is a cause of disease Y but what matters most for health and how we can best achieve public health goals.

In this chapter, we aim to concretize this approach and to explore how we may engage a consequentialist epidemiology that considers what matters most. To do so, first we review the seven steps of an epidemiologic study that formed the backbone of this book. We then apply those seven steps around three issues that we think are paramount to any consideration of a consequential epidemiology: the trade-off between comparability and external validity, the concept of small effects translating to large improvements in population health, and the global context of health and disease.

Revisited: The Seven Steps of an Epidemiologic Study of Consequence

In this book we have guided the reader through seven steps that we can use to design, analyze, and draw inference from epidemiologic studies. First, we conceptualize a population of interest, setting specific eligibility criteria that may be defined by time and place, specific characteristics of individuals, and/or factors that promote a successful study. Second, we conceptualize health indicators and exposures that are of interest to our goal of improving the population's health and we create reliable and valid measures that reflect the underlying constructs. Third, we take a sample of that population. Depending on the goal of the study, we may take a representative sample or construct a purposive sample to maximize the comparability between groups. Fourth, we estimate measures of association for the effect of an exposure on a health indicator, ruling out with some degree of confidence that the result documented could have arisen by chance in the sampling process. Fifth, we rigorously test that association to determine whether the association reflects a causal association. As a sixth step, we assess the potential factors that may, jointly with the exposure of interest, also cause disease. Therefore, we assess the extent to which component causes in the same sufficient cause modify the association of interest within the study sample by estimating measures of interaction. And finally, as a seventh step, we assess the extent to which the result is externally valid to other populations by assessing the prevalence of causal partners of the exposure of interest across populations. Further, although it is not a specific step in conducting an epidemiologic study, an eye toward early prevention and intervention is a necessary foundation of epidemiology; thus, understanding concepts in screening is critical to implementing our science for public health improvement.

Although these steps provide an overview of the foundational methods that underlie our science, we note that epidemiologic methods are an active area of research and development. The reader who is taking upper-level epidemiologic courses will undoubtedly encounter many of these emerging methods. We would expect that this highly generative area of research will—in coming decades—lead to both refinement and perhaps rethinking of some of the dominant approaches in the field that we discuss here.

Balancing the Demands of Comparability and External Validity

As we have detailed throughout this book, there are many reasons to conduct an epidemiologic study, and many questions that can be answered with such studies. Indeed, there are so many questions that we can well lose sight of why we are doing the study to begin with. It is with that in mind that we conclude the book with a call for clarity of purpose. To our mind, all epidemiologic studies should be conducted with a clear intent to improve the health of populations. We are well aware, of course, that no one study can stand alone without an evidence base. However, that recognition does not absolve us of our responsibility to carefully interrogate why we are conducting a particular study and how any given study contributes to the larger overall effort that aims to identify causes so that we may act and improve population health.

In Chapter 1, we articulated a vision for population health that required us to ask questions beyond how and why individuals become ill and instead how and why some groups become more ill than other groups. In Chapter 2 we invoked the classic example by Geoffrey Rose discussing the observation that causes of risk in one group versus another may be distinct (yet related to and ultimately embedded within) causes of individual cases, and that an epidemiologic approach to public health requires us to conceptualize the health of populations and intervene to shift the curve of population health by focusing on the identification of factors that shape the health of entire groups or populations (Rose, 1985). Rose articulates the notion that our studies should have consequence for populations and population health. For our studies to have consequence, we must consider not only the primacy of identifying causal effects but also the external validity of these effects of the results from our study sample when they are applied to the population in its complex reality.

This concept, beguiling in its simplicity, embeds substantial challenges for the field. Consistent with this, in our teaching and practice, we have found that there are two central elements of epidemiologic study design—comparability and external validity—that inevitably need to be grappled with if we have consequentialist goals in mind.

We have discussed throughout this book how we attempt to achieve comparability within our study sample such that we can determine causal effect estimates that are internally valid. In particular, in Chapter 10, we described randomization, matching, and stratification as foundational approaches to attempt comparability within a study sample. The challenge arises in choosing samples that allow us to maximize comparability between exposed and unexposed. More often than not, epidemiologic studies are based on purposive samples. A purposive sample that achieves comparability through careful eligibility criteria as well as randomization of exposure can provide unparalleled insights into the etiology of disease. In fact, such studies are necessary so that we can provide rigorous estimation of the causal effects of various exposures on important outcomes. However, purposive samples almost inevitably challenge our capacity to study a population whose characteristics compare to those of the population on which we aim to intervene. This sets up the challenge—obtaining an internally valid estimate through a sample with perfect comparability is meaningless if the causal estimate obtained does not apply in the specific population to which we would like to intervene.

We have also discussed throughout this book the conditions under which a specific causal effect applies across populations. First, in Chapter 7, we described how most causes of disease do not act in isolation; they require a constellation of additional causes that together produce disease. The process of causes acting together to produce disease is termed interaction. In the language we developed in Chapter 7, we would say that interaction occurs when two marbles are both needed to fill a specific marble jar. If two causes interact, then both causes are necessary (marbles) as part of that sufficient cause (marble jar) for the health indicator to occur through that sufficient cause. In Chapter 11, we formalized the process of assessing interaction in our data; interaction is evident when the risk of disease among those exposed to two potential causes is greater than the sum of their individual effects. Then, in Chapter 12, we described how a particular relation between an exposure and a health indicator from a study sample will be externally valid to another population to the extent that the causes that interact with the exposure (other marbles in the same marble jars) are distributed similarly between the study sample and the population to which we wish to infer.

Thus, given this base of knowledge, it is evident that understanding the factors that are involved in producing a causal estimate is critical to the conduct of epidemiologic studies that matter for the population of interest. This does not in any way lessen the importance of comparability between the exposed and the unexposed. In many cases, the insights gained from a sample with good comparability will be externally valid well beyond the study sample even if the study sample is not explicitly designed to represent the population on which we would like to intervene (Rothman, Gallacher, & Hatch, 2013). However, at the core, a tension remains. Our efforts to maximize internal validity through comparability pushes us to choose samples where we can ensure comparability, often at the expense of external validity of the sample.

Small Effects, Big Implications

One central consideration for those who are interested in a consequential epidemiology is whether the effect obtained in the epidemiologic study has consequence for the populations in which burden of disease is greatest. A second question that is central here is whether the effect estimates obtained in our studies translate into actual cases of illness and disease that may be prevented through public health action. When considering such questions, the magnitude of the estimate of effect must be conceptualized within the context of the prevalence of the exposure of interest itself. That is, exposure–health indicator relations for which there is a small magnitude of effect may in fact translate to large public health benefits.

Consider the following example. We are interested in intervening to prevent the occurrence of a particular disease in Farrlandia, which has an overall population risk of about 6 per 100 over a 5-year period. There are two exposures in the population that have well-documented associations with disease: Exposure A is associated with an increased 1.2 times greater risk for the onset of the disease, and Exposure B is associated with a fivefold increase in the risk of disease. Which exposure should we invest public health time and money in preventing? Based on the risk ratio, we may initially conclude Exposure B, as the relation between exposure and outcome is stronger for Exposure B compared with Exposure A. However, when we consider public health intervention in terms of the population health impact, we realize that the answer may depend in some part on the prevalence of each of these exposures. Tables 14.1 and 14.2 display the 2 × 2 table of the association between Exposure A and disease (Table 14.1) and Exposure B and disease (Table 14.2).

Table 14.1 Expected Occurrence of Disease Over 5 Years Based
on Exposure A

	Disease	No Disease	Total
Exposed to A	48	752	800
Unexposed to A	10	190	200
Total	58	942	1,000
5-year risk	58/1,000 = 0.058		
Risk ratio	$(48/800)/(10/200) = 1.20$		
Risk difference	$(48/800) - (10/200) = 0.010$		

Exposure A has a prevalence of 80% (800/1,000) in the population of interest. With an expected risk ratio of 1.2 and an overall 5-year risk of about 6%, we would expect to observe the data in Table 14.1 in a population of 1,000 Farrlandians. We have 48 individuals who were both exposed to A and developed the disease. Assuming that about 6% of these individuals would have developed the disease even in the absence of exposure to A (about 3 cases), and assuming complete comparability between exposed and unexposed individuals, we conclude that Exposure to A caused about 45 cases of disease.

Exposure B has a prevalence of 5% in the population of interest (50/1,000). With an expected risk ratio of 5.0 and the same overall 6% expected 5-year risk, we turn toward Table 14.2 to see the data we would expect to observe. There are 13 individuals that are both exposed to B and who develop the disease. Again assuming that about 6% of these individuals would have developed the disease even in the absence of exposure to A (about 1 case) and

Table 14.2 Expected Occurrence of Disease Over 5 Years Based
on Exposure B

	Disease	No Disease	Total
Exposed to B	13	37	50
Unexposed to B	48	902	950
Total	61	939	1,000
5-year risk	61/1000 = 0.061		
Risk ratio	$(13/50)/(48/902) = 5.15$		
Risk difference	$(13/50) - (48/902) = 0.21$		

complete comparability between exposed and unexposed, we conclude that Exposure to B caused about 12 cases of disease.

Thus, even though Exposure to A has a weaker overall effect on disease compared with Exposure B, it is responsible for almost four times more cases than Exposure B because it is so much more prevalent in the population.

When considering how to move beyond the identification of true causes of adverse health in populations to intervention that reduce disease in populations, considerations of scope and distribution of exposures must be considered. At the most extreme, ubiquitous exposures are almost certainly important by virtue of their high prevalence. Therefore, for example, particulate air pollution—to which millions are exposed—has been shown to have substantial impact on the risk of cardiovascular disease in a population, including out of hospital cardiac arrests, despite relatively low measures of association between the exposure and the disease (Teng et al., 2013). Such observations have contributed to measures to curb air pollution worldwide.

Public health resources must compete with other societal resource expenditures. Therefore, decisions we make about public health resource allocation are not cost free. A focus on rare exposures with high magnitudes of association with disease outcomes may yield few public health wins, whereas a focus on common exposures with small overall effects may have a larger impact on public health. Although reduction in exposure to any cause of adverse human health is important, a consequentialist approach to epidemiology requires us to consider our research questions and the conduct of epidemiology through the lens of the exposures that will produce the greatest impact on human health.

The Local and the Global Implications of Consequentialist Epidemiology

There are many uses for public health and epidemiology. Public health is traditionally a community health science. But what is a community, and are the borders of our communities changing? Epidemiologists engaged in local public health efforts may be explicitly interested in understanding the local ecology of health in a particular village, city, state, or country; describing the health conditions that affect a specific population of interest; and intervening to reduce the incidence and improve the outcomes of those conditions. Other epidemiologists are engaged in a more universal goal—to understand the causes of human disease more generally and to improve the health of the populations for whom the burden of disease is greatest. Although we are inevitably interested in the health of local populations, asking questions about what matters for population health forces us to design studies that have broader implications. In other words, asking a research question that truly matters for the health of populations can change the scope of what we are examining.

Acknowledging that health is not distributed equally across populations, an epidemiology of consequence must engage in science well beyond local borders. Consider the data on mortality per 1,000 live births across country. Early childhood mortality rates are often used as a benchmark for the health of a country and the efficacy of health systems because mortality in children is often preventable and/or amenable with effective intervention and care. In Figure 14.1, we show the mortality rate per 1,000 live births in 12 countries (United Nations Inter-agency Group for Child Mortality Estimation, 2012). Within these 12 countries, the United States is performing the worst, with slightly more than 7 deaths per 1,000 live births. The fact that the United States underperforms other high-income countries with respect to health has been well documented, and the necessity of research on reasons for this underperformance has received increasing attention (Woolf & Aron, 2013). However, examine the panel on the bottom in Figure 14.1, with the child mortality rate in Ethiopia added. Differences among the high-income countries are now barely discernible given that the child mortality rate in Ethiopia is more than 17 times higher than in the United States.

We have articulated a framework for elucidating the causes of child mortality in this book. If we conduct a study in the United States, we would take a sample of the population (Chapter 4), measure the potential causes of greatest interest (Chapter 5), estimate associations for the effect of those potential causes on child mortality (Chapter 6), rigorously assess those associations for internal validity (Chapters 8 through 10), and consider the potential factors that activate causes through assessment of interaction (Chapter 11). We have also described how the causes of child mortality among those in one population (e.g., the United States) may not be the same as the causes of child mortality in another population (e.g., Ethiopia) and that we must carefully consider the conditions under which the results from one population would be externally valid across populations (Chapter 12). As Rose (1985) articulates, the causes of child mortality in the United States may be different than the causes of the extreme disparity in child mortality between the United States and Ethiopia. Beyond these considerations, however, there is the larger question of what we study and among whom.

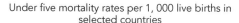

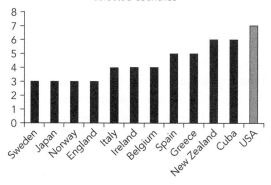

Mortality rate, under-5 (per 1,000 live births). The World Bank Data, 2012. United Nations Inter-agency Group for Child Mortality Estimation (UNICEF, WHO, World Bank, UN DESA Population Division). <http://data.worldbank.org/indicator/SH.DYN.MORT> Accessed October 29, 2013.

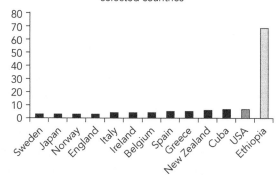

Mortality rate, under-5 (per 1,000 live births). The World Bank Data, 2012. United Nations Inter-agency Group for Child Mortality Estimation (UNICEF, WHO, World Bank, UN DESA Population Division). <http://data.worldbank.org/indicator/SH.DYN.MORT> Accessed October 29, 2013.

FIGURE 14.1 Under age 5 mortality rate per 1,000 live births in 12 countries (top), and including Ethiopia (bottom).

An epidemiology of consequence must acknowledge that the pressing public health issues of our time require a broad, global viewpoint that maximizes the potential for improving the health of all populations. Although child mortality in any country should be studied with an eye toward reduction, these figures make clear that an epidemiological research agenda that purports to improve population health may achieve a greater improvement in population health, globally, with a focus on understanding the causes of mortality in resource-poor versus resource-rich settings.

Uncovering the determinants of human disease is a stirring scientific goal, yet these determinants are often context specific and may translate into many cases of disease or a few cases of disease depending on the overall burden on health and the distribution of other causes of disease that share a marble jar with specific causes of interest. A globally focused epidemiologic practice that encourages inquiry into the settings, exposures, and outcomes contributing to the greatest burden across populations is central to ensuring that our science lives up to the ideals of disease prevention and population health promotion goals. Further, a broad scope of inquiry that focuses less on investigating causes of disease within populations and instead asks difficult yet necessary questions about why some populations have higher burdens than other populations is likely to yield epidemiologic findings that translate into demonstrable wins for public health practice and intervention efforts.

Causal Explanation Versus Intervention

Challenging our efforts to engage in a consequential epidemiology, the effects of causes are not necessarily equal to the effects of interventions on those causes (Schwartz, Gatto, & Campbell, 2011). In epidemiologic studies we isolate the specific effects of exposures of interest by creating comparable exposed and unexposed groups. Although a perfectly designed epidemiologic study with complete comparability can give us a measure of the total number of cases that could be prevented by removing the exposure of interest ceteris paribus, the actual process of removing the exposure of interest cannot be done in isolation. Prevention efforts will not likely be complete in removing all of the exposure, and may have unintended consequences that could increase adverse health of another outcome, change the distribution of component causes in such a way that adverse health remains, or have an even larger (or smaller) effect on the health indicator than was expected given the observed causal effect of the exposure. Efforts have been made in epidemiology in recent years to expand capacity and expertise in mathematical simulation modeling to understand the potential unintended and downstream consequences of health interventions (Galea, Riddle, & Kaplan, 2010). Such efforts are critical to moving from the identification of causes of adverse health to understanding the implications of intervening on the causes that have been identified.

Summary

Epidemiologic research has been the cornerstone of public health science for centuries. Our goal in this book was to provide the introductory epidemiology student with an overview of the foundational methods of epidemiology, aiming to equip students with the tools to design, execute, and evaluate epidemiologic studies that can contribute to improvements in population health in decades to come. This book, as must all introductory textbooks, sits self-consciously on the shoulders of many other books and contributions to the field that have preceded it. However, we have also in this book adopted a particular approach, informed by our understanding of the foundations of the field and by our concern with contributing to an epidemiology of consequence. Therefore, we have aimed to induct the reader into an appreciation of the concepts that underlie epidemiologic principles, starting with an understanding of populations and helping the reader develop an intuition about how we may measure exposures and health indicators within those populations. We then moved on to how we may take a population sample before exploring how we may assess causes in that sample, both working in isolation and together with other causes as part of complex causal structures. We hope, in adopting this approach, that the student who is taking only one epidemiology course in his or her career can retain an appreciation of the foundations of the discipline, leaving with a lifetime appreciation for the possibilities, and challenges, facing efforts to improve population health. We hope that for the student who will go on to take upper level epidemiology courses, this book provides a primer on how to think about epidemiology that will serve well as preparation for deeper engagement with the science of population health.

References

Galea, S. (2013). An argument for a consequentialist epidemiology. *American Journal of Epidemiology, 178*, 1185–1191.

Galea, S., Riddle, M., & Kaplan, G. A. (2010). Causal thinking and complex system approaches in epidemiology. *International Journal of Epidemiology, 39*, 97–106.

Rose, G. (1985). Sick individuals and sick populations. *International Journal of Epidemiology, 14*, 32–38.

Rothman, K. J., Gallacher, J. E., & Hatch, E. E. (2013). Why representativeness should be avoided. *International Journal of Epidemiology, 42*, 1012–1014.

Schwartz, S., Gatto, N., & Campbell, U. (2011). What would have been is not what would be: Counterfactuals of the past and potential outcomes of the future. In P. Shrout,

K. Keyes, & K. Ornstein (Eds.), *Causality and psychopathology*. New York: Oxford University Press.

Teng, T. H., Williams, T. A., Bremner, A., Tohira, H., Franklin, P., Tonkin, A., . . . Finn, J. (2013). A systematic review of air pollution and incidence of out-of-hospital cardiac arrest. *Journal of Epidemiology & Community Health*, *68*, 37–43.

United Nations Inter-agency Group for Child Mortality Estimation (UNICEF, WHO, World Bank, UN DESA Population Division). (2012). Mortality rate, under-5 (per 1,000 live births). The World Bank Data, 2012.

Woolf, S. H., & Aron, L. (2013). *U.S. health in international perspective: Shorter lives, poorer health*. Washington, DC: Institute of Medicine of the National Academies.

Index